CARLAT PUBLISHING

GERIATRIC PSYCHIATRY FACT BOOK

FIRST EDITION

Rehan Aziz, MD

Program Director
Psychiatry Residency Program
Jersey Shore University Medical Center

Associate Program Director
Geriatric Psychiatry Fellowship Program
Jersey Shore University Medical Center

Associate Professor of Psychiatry and Neurology
Hackensack Meridian School of Medicine

Published by Carlat Publishing, LLC
PO Box 626, Newburyport, MA 01950

CARLAT PUBLISHING

Geriatric Psychiatry Fact Book

FIRST EDITION

Published by Carlat Publishing, LLC
PO Box 626, Newburyport, MA 01950

Publisher and Editor-in-Chief: Daniel J. Carlat, MD
Deputy Editor: Talia Puzantian, PharmD, BCPP
Senior Editor: Ilana Fogelson

This CME/CE activity is intended for psychiatrists, psychiatric nurses, psychologists, and other health care professionals with an interest in mental health. The Carlat CME Institute is accredited by the Accreditation Council for Continuing Medical Education to provide continuing medical education for physicians. Carlat CME Institute maintains responsibility for this program and its content. Carlat CME Institute designates this enduring material educational activity for a maximum of twelve [12] AMA PRA Category 1 Credits™. Physicians or psychologists should claim credit commensurate only with the extent of their participation in the activity. The American Board of Psychiatry and Neurology has reviewed the *Geriatric Psychiatry Fact Book* and has approved this program as part of a comprehensive Self-Assessment and CME Program, which is mandated by ABMS as a necessary component of maintenance of certification. CME tests must be taken online at www.thecarlatreport.com/cme (for ABPN SA course subscribers).

To order, visit www.thecarlatreport.com
or call (866) 348-9279

ISBN #:
Print: 979-8-9893264-4-0
eBook: 979-8-9893264-5-7

PRINTED IN THE UNITED STATES OF AMERICA

With deepest gratitude to Sarah, Layla, Jasim, Nyla, Sylvie, and Evee—without whom this work couldn't have been written. Their unwavering patience, love, and belief in this project have been my constant source of motivation.

Table of Contents

List of Tables

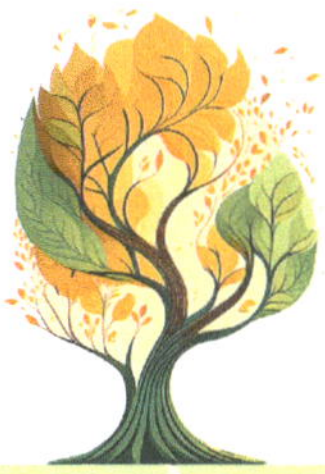

Introduction to Geriatric Psychiatry

Over the course of my career, I've had the privilege of working with countless older adults and their families. These experiences have profoundly shaped my understanding of mental health and the aging process. What I've learned is that treating older patients requires honoring their resilience, listening to their stories, collaborating with their families, and appreciating the wisdom they've accumulated through decades of lived experience.

Effective clinical practice in geriatric psychiatry demands a sophisticated understanding of the complex interplay between the biological vulnerabilities, psychological stressors, and sociocultural contexts that uniquely influence mental health in later life. Older adults also navigate significant life transitions like retirement, bereavement, chronic illness, and cognitive changes, while often depending on support networks. The geriatrician must consider all these factors to deliver truly exceptional care.

As our population ages, the need for specialized expertise in geriatric psychiatry has never been greater. Yet, we face a critical shortage of practitioners equipped with the necessary skills and knowledge in this field. This book addresses this gap by offering evidence-based, high-yield clinical insights accessible at the point of care. My goal is to empower a broad range of health care professionals with the tools to provide competent, compassionate care to older adults that takes into account the unique challenges they face. At some point, most older adults will require some form of community support; thus, to supplement this text, I've also compiled valuable resources for clinical practice, available at the end of this book.

The process of writing this book has been a labor of love. The opportunity to contribute to a resource that can enhance patient care is profoundly fulfilling. Above all, I remain continually inspired by the resilience, dignity, and wisdom of the older adults we serve, whose experiences provide enduring lessons in humanity and compassion. Lessons that I hope will inspire your practice as they have mine.

Geriatric Assessment

Psychiatric Assessment of Older Adults

The psychiatric assessment of older adults builds upon standard adult evaluation practices but includes special attention to age-related factors. In this section, I'll walk you through key modifications and additional elements to consider when evaluating older patients.

CLINICAL PEARL: *Always involve a family member or caregiver in the assessment when possible. They often provide crucial information about functional changes that the patient may not recognize or report.*

Style and Technique

Many older adults experience hearing loss. This can cause them to feel left out of appointments or have difficulty understanding questions. I've found these techniques particularly helpful:

- Face the patient and talk clearly and slowly.
- Speak a little louder than usual without shouting.
- Repeat yourself as needed.
- Direct your voice to the ear with better hearing.
- Use gestures or facial expressions to get your points across.
- Provide written materials that the patient can refer to later.
- Consider the room setup—minimize background noise and ensure good lighting.

PRACTICE POINT: *If you suspect hearing difficulties, ask "With which ear do you hear better?" at the start of the session. This simple question can dramatically improve communication.*

Chief Complaint

Begin by recording the patient's main concern in their own words. This provides valuable insight into the patient's perspective and helps prioritize their needs.

History of Presenting Illness (HPI)

In addition to the standard HPI questions, when conducting psychiatric evaluations in older adults, it is essential to assess functional and cognitive status. This practice ensures a comprehensive evaluation, enabling accurate diagnosis and management plans tailored to the unique needs of older patients. (See "Functional Assessment in Older Adults" [page 12] and "Neurocognitive Testing for Dementia" [page 101] fact sheets in the "Geriatric Assessment" and "Assessment and Treatment of Neurocognitive Disorders" sections of this book.)

Here are some pointers on cognitive domains to assess in older adults and how responses may guide clinical interpretation:

Memory changes

Short-term memory typically declines before long-term memory in conditions like Alzheimer's dementia (AD). Ask:

- "Have you noticed any changes in your memory or have you become more forgetful?"
- "How is your memory for recent events?"
- "Have you been forgetting appointments, birthdays, or anniversaries?
- "Have you lost or misplaced items like your keys, purse, or wallet?"
- "How is your memory for things that happened a long time ago?"

CLINICAL PEARL: *Pay attention to how patients answer these questions. Do they turn to their family member to confirm details? Do they seem embarrassed or frustrated? These observations can be very telling.*

Attention and processing speed

These domains often decline together and can significantly impact daily functioning. I find it helpful to both ask questions and observe behavior during the interview:

- "Do you have trouble following conversations or TV shows?"
- "Does your thinking feel slower than it used to?"
- "Do you need more time to make decisions?"

Language

Listen for issues with word-finding, grammar, naming, and word substitutions. Deficits in grammar and word-finding can be seen in language-specific forms of AD and frontotemporal dementia (FTD). Ask:

- "Do you have trouble finding the right words?"
- "Are you forgetting the names of things?"

Visuospatial function

Losses here might result in the inability to navigate in familiar environments or judge distances. Difficulty with three-dimensional relationships could suggest AD or dementia with Lewy bodies (DLB), though also ask your patient about their vision.

- "Have you been getting lost in familiar places or been found wandering?"
- "Do you restrict your driving to nearby areas or only to daylight hours?"

Thinking/reasoning

Trouble with reasoning is found early on in FTD and later in AD and other dementias. Ask about higher-level critical thinking and problem-solving skills:

- "Are you having trouble following storylines in movies or books?"
- "Are you having trouble making decisions?"

Social comportment

This can be impaired initially in FTD and, along with early personality change, is a mark of the disease. It can also be altered in a specific form of AD that targets the frontal lobes. Patients are often unaware of their faux pas. Ask the older adult's family:

- "Has there been any inappropriate behavior or comments in public?"
- "Has their personality changed?"

Behavioral symptoms

I've found it crucial to assess for behavioral changes, as they often accompany cognitive decline. These symptoms frequently cause more distress than the memory problems. Ask about:

- Aggression
- Agitation
- Apathy
- Depression
- Resistance to care
- Sundowning (increased confusion in the evening and night hours)

PRACTICE POINT: *Always ask about sundowning specifically—many families do not volunteer this information because they assume it is normal aging.*

Getting collateral information

In geriatric psychiatry, collateral information is not just helpful—it is essential. I always try to:

- Obtain consent to speak with family members or include them in the process itself, though in these situations, it is important to ensure that the patient gets their say.
- Ask caregivers about:
  - Symptom progression
  - Changes in daily routine
  - Social withdrawal
  - Safety concerns
  - Medication administration
  - Financial management

Psychiatric Review of Systems

If not already covered in the history of presenting illness, ask additional screening questions, based on your level of suspicion, for the following:

- Anxiety
- Bipolar disorder (including mania or hypomania)
- Depression
- Psychosis
- Somatic disorders (including eating disorders and somatic symptom disorder)
- Substance use

Past Psychiatric History

- *Prior diagnoses:* Ask about any previously diagnosed psychiatric conditions.
- *Psychiatric hospitalizations:* Note the number, dates, duration, and reasons for any hospitalizations.
- *Medication trials:* Obtain details on psychotropic medications previously prescribed, their effectiveness, side effects, and reasons for discontinuation. Also ask about any history of electroconvulsive therapy (ECT), transcranial magnetic stimulation (TMS), or esketamine treatment.
- *Psychotherapy:* Ask about types of therapy received (eg, cognitive behavioral therapy [CBT], dialectical behavior therapy [DBT], psychodynamic, group), frequency, and duration, along with their effectiveness.
- *Suicide attempts:* Record any history of suicide attempts, including methods and circumstances.

- *Self-harm behaviors:* Inquire about behaviors such as cutting, burning, or scratching, as well as frequency and triggers.
- *Trauma history:* Ask about any significant trauma, such as physical, emotional, or sexual abuse, as well as its impact on the patient.
- *Outpatient providers:* Ascertain the patient's current and past mental health providers, their specialties, and duration of care. Obtain permission to contact these providers for collateral history.

Substance Use History

- Always inquire about the use of nicotine, alcohol, illicit substances (eg, cocaine, heroin), and prescription drug misuse.
- Note that substance use rates have increased among older adults due to the aging baby boomer population and increased legalization of marijuana.
- Older adults are more likely to misuse prescription medications than use illicit substances.
- If substance misuse is reported, gather specific details, including:
  - Types of substances used
  - Frequency and quantity of use
  - Most recent use
  - History of withdrawal symptoms (eg, delirium tremens, seizures)
  - Complications from use (eg, cognitive impairment, falls, liver disease)
  - History of rehabilitation programs, such as:
    - Inpatient or outpatient treatment
    - Participation in Alcoholics Anonymous or Narcotics Anonymous

Past Medical History

Physical health

Maintaining a healthy lifestyle and effectively managing chronic conditions helps older adults maintain independence. Ask: "Have you experienced any issues with your health, vision, hearing, teeth, or had any recent falls?"

Medical conditions

Inquire about the presence of the following conditions, as they may contribute to or exacerbate psychiatric symptoms as well as cognitive impairment.

- Cardiovascular disease
- Diabetes
- Head injuries
- Metabolic abnormalities
- Neurological illnesses (eg, strokes, seizures, Parkinson's disease)
- Pulmonary disease
- Thyroid disorders

Sensory function

- *Vision and hearing*
  - Impaired vision and hearing can reduce independence, contribute to social isolation, and increase the risk of dementia and depression.
  - Refer patients to an audiologist for a hearing evaluation or to an ophthalmologist/optometrist for a vision assessment as needed.
- *Smell loss*
  - Loss of the sense of smell may be an early sign of neurodegenerative disease.
- *Dental health*
  - Poor dental hygiene is associated with major neurocognitive disorder. Inquire about patients' dental habits and encourage regular dental visits.
- *Falls*
  - One-third of older adults experience at least one fall annually, and 20% of falls result in an injury.
  - Evaluate the frequency of falls and identify underlying causes and contributing factors.
  - Falls can lead to a decline in functional status, reduced participation in social activities, and diminished quality of life.

CLINICAL PEARL: *Always ask "What medical conditions affect your daily life the most?" This often reveals different priorities than what may be listed in the medical record.*

Medications

- *Investigate all products*: Since many older adults use over-the-counter medications, herbal supplements, and vitamins, engage in a thorough discussion of these agents.
- *Review current medications*: Evaluate all prescribed medications for potential drug interactions or side effects that might impair psychological, cognitive, or physical functioning.
- *Assess medication appropriateness*: Determine the necessity and suitability of each medication within the context of the patient's overall health and treatment goals.
- *Be cautious of polypharmacy*: Monitor for polypharmacy and avoid drugs with anticholinergic properties, as both can exacerbate cognitive impairment.
- *Coordinate with primary care provider (PCP)*: If a reconciliation reveals no clear rationale for a non-psychotropic medication that may be harmful, consider reaching out to the patient's PCP for further clarification.

Allergies and Adverse Reactions

When inquiring, create a distinction among:

- *True allergies*: Immune-mediated responses such as anaphylaxis, angioedema, or urticaria.
- *Intolerance*: Nonimmune symptoms like gastrointestinal upset or mild discomfort.
- *Adverse reactions*: Side effects, such as sedation or dizziness.

Family Psychiatric History

- Ask about a family history of psychiatric disorders, substance use disorders, and deaths from suicide.
- Inquire about any family history of dementia or AD, specifically noting the age of onset.

Social History

- *Chronological approach*
  - Begin with the patient's early life, including birthplace and family composition.
  - Educational background: Highest level of education achieved.
  - Employment history:
    - Past occupations, employment status, and current income source.
    - Assess for financial difficulties that may impact access to food, medication, or healthcare.
  - Relationship history: Marital status, history of significant relationships, and children (including their level of involvement in the patient's care).
  - Current living conditions:
    - Determine whether the patient resides alone or with others, and if so, who those individuals are.
    - If in a facility, inquire about the level of care and satisfaction with the living environment.
  - Legal and military history: Ask about any history of legal involvement or military service, including access to veteran's benefits.
- *Advance care planning*
  - Key questions:
    - Does the patient have a living will, power of attorney, or guardian?
    - If these documents are not in place, suggest a referral to an elder law attorney to assist with future planning.
- *Caregiver information*
  - Role of social supports:
    - Social supports significantly influence mental health, functional independence, and quality of life in older adults. Inquire about the patient's network, including partners, children, relatives, or friends who can assist with tasks like finances, transportation, meals, medications, or household chores.
  - Key questions:
    - "Whom do you turn to when you need help with personal or medical issues?"
    - "Whom would you call in an emergency?"
    - "Do you receive any help at home, such as a home companion, home health aide, visiting nurse, or housekeeper?"
  - Evaluating support adequacy:
    - Ask: "During the past few weeks, was someone available if you needed or wanted help?"
- *Social engagement*
  - Community involvement: Inquire about the patient's participation in activities like senior centers, religious gatherings, hobby clubs, and volunteer programs.
  - Maintaining relationships: Ask how the patient keeps in touch with family and friends to assess for potential social isolation.

Functional Assessment in Older Adults

Evaluating functional status helps identify specific activities for which an older adult needs assistance and determine appropriate support levels. But this assessment is not just about checking boxes—it is about understanding how deficits impact quality of life and safety. When I identify concerns, I first consider whether they can be addressed through adaptive equipment, home modifications, or additional community support before recommending more restrictive care settings.

Functional impairment is also a key criterion for diagnosing dementia, making this assessment crucial for diagnosis and care planning. To assess functional capacity, I focus on two main areas: **1)** basic activities of daily living (ADLs) and **2)** instrumental activities of daily living (IADLs). IADLs are more complex skills that typically decline first in dementia, while ADLs are basic self-care tasks often affected in the moderate to severe stages. I find it is essential to conduct this assessment with a caregiver present, as patients may be unaware of or minimize their deficits.

The table at the end of this fact sheet describes two helpful (if somewhat morbid) mnemonics to help you remember these questions—DEATH and SHAFT.

CLINICAL PEARL: *The pattern of functional loss often suggests specific conditions. Isolated IADL decline with preserved ADLs may indicate early dementia, while simultaneous decline in both often suggests medical illness or depression.*

In most cases, patients with IADL impairments can manage in the community with increased support. Some may benefit from transitioning to senior housing or assisted living. Those with significant ADL impairments typically need more substantial care, either through intensive family support or at a skilled nursing facility.

Instrumental Activities of Daily Living

Impairment in IADLs can signal underlying cognitive issues, such as problems with memory, judgment, or problem-solving. While some cognitive decline is normal with aging, significant loss requires a thorough evaluation. I start with: "Are you having trouble carrying out your usual daily activities?" Then I explore specific areas:

- *Shopping*
  - "Do you shop for groceries or other necessities by yourself?"
  - "Do you find yourself using shopping lists more frequently?"
  - "Do you sometimes forget essential items or end up buying things you don't need?"
- *Housekeeping*
  - "Have you noticed any changes or difficulties in managing household chores?"
  - "Are you able to sweep, vacuum, or mop the floors independently?"
- *Accounting*
  - "Are you comfortable handling money, paying by credit/debit card, or writing checks independently?"
  - "Have you double paid or incurred late fees?"
  - "Have you fallen for any scams?"
- *Food preparation*
  - "Are you able to prepare your meals independently?"
  - "Have you experienced any recent kitchen accidents, eg, burning food, leaving stove unattended?"
  - "Are you having difficulty following recipes or cooking instructions?"
- *Transportation*
  - "Do you drive?" If yes, "Have you been in any accidents over the past year?"
  - "Have you had problems identifying landmarks or signs?"
  - "Have you driven without a seat belt?"
  - "Are you driving less on the freeway, closer to home, or only during the day" (Chee JN et al, *Am J Geriatr Psychiatry* 2017;25(12):1376-1390)?
- *Additional:* Inquire about difficulty using computers, cell phones, electronics, and taking medications.
  - For meds, ask, "Do you ever forget to take your medications? Do you use a pill box or organizer? Does anyone help you manage or set up your medications?"

Basic Activities of Daily Living

ADLs focus on fundamental physical tasks like bathing, dressing, and eating. Difficulty with ADLs typically emerges in the later stages of dementia. Caregivers are often the first to notice these changes and should be included in the assessment process. If the patient experiences falls, choking, or incontinence, refer them to their primary care physician for a comprehensive evaluation.

- *Dressing*
  - "Do you need help getting dressed?"
  - "Have you worn clothes inside out or had trouble with buttons?"
- *Eating*
  - "Have you been eating more sweets or carbs?"
    - Carbohydrate craving can also occur in the early stages of frontotemporal dementia.
  - "Have you had any trouble cutting food, using forks/knives/spoons, eating, or swallowing?"
- *Ambulating*
  - "Have you had any falls in the last six months"?
  - If so, "What caused them?"
- *Toileting*
  - "Have you had any bathroom accidents?
  - "Have you started using adult diapers or incontinence pads?"
- *Hygiene*
  - "How often are you bathing?"
    - Many older adults with dementia become resistant to showering.
  - "Have you had any difficulty with using hot or cold knobs or applying soap?"
  - "Have you had trouble brushing your teeth or combing your hair?"

Table 1: **DEATH and SHAFT Mnemonics for Geriatric Functional Assessment**

ADLs[1]	IADLs[1]
Dressing "Have you needed help getting dressed?"	**Shopping** • "How do you typically shop for groceries and personal items?" • "Have you had trouble handling money or credit cards?"
Eating "Do you need assistance with your meals?"	**Housekeeping** • "Are you having trouble keeping your living area clean?" • "Do you have difficulty operating the dishwasher or doing the laundry?"
Ambulating • "Do you experience trouble getting out of bed or a chair?" • "How many falls have you had in the past few months?"	**Accounting** "How do you keep up with finances and bills?"
Toileting "Do you have difficulty getting to the bathroom in time? Have you had accidents?"	**Food Preparation** • "How do you manage your meals?" • "Do you cook for yourself?" • "Have you burned food or left the stove/oven unattended?"
Hygiene • "Do you need assistance bathing?" • "Do you need help combing your hair or brushing your teeth?"	**Transportation** • "Have you gotten lost while driving?" • "Have you been in any accidents in the last year?"

[1] *Source: Bickley LS.* Bates' Guide to Physical Examination and History Taking. *12th ed. Alphen aan den Rign, The Netherlands: Wolters Kluwer; 2017.*

Physical Exam and Laboratory Testing in Geriatric Psychiatry

The physical exam and laboratory testing are especially important in geriatric psychiatry because medical conditions or medications often trigger psychiatric symptoms. This fact sheet focuses on key elements that psychiatrists should feel comfortable performing, while ensuring patients maintain regular care with their primary care physicians.

CLINICAL PEARL: *Even subtle changes in physical health can cause significant psychiatric symptoms in older adults. I have found that a systematic approach to the exam helps catch these shifts early.*

Physical Exam

Vital signs

- Record blood pressure, heart rate, respiratory rate, and temperature.
- Fluctuations can be influenced by common medications, like antipsychotics or antidepressants, which may affect cardiovascular or thermoregulatory systems.

General appearance

- Observe general state, including personal hygiene and grooming (poor grooming can be a sign of a deteriorating mental state, cognitive decline, or elder abuse).
- Note any behaviors indicative of anxiety (nervous), depression (withdrawn), or psychosis (apprehensive or distracted by internal stimuli).

Neurological system

- Assess for movement disorders, in particular rigidity or tremors, which could be side effects of antipsychotic medications or due to Parkinson's disease (PD).
  - Patients with PD often exhibit an upper extremity "pill-rolling" tremor that appears when their arms are relaxed. Other characteristic PD signs are lack of facial expression, decreased arm swing, stooped posture, slowed movements, and shuffling steps when walking.
  - Essential tremor (ET) is another common disorder in older adults. In contrast to PD, ET occurs when muscles are voluntarily contracted to maintain a posture, like when holding a cup, or when performing other movements.

CLINICAL PEARL: *A short, shuffling gait may suggest parkinsonism as a side effect of antipsychotic medications but consider normal pressure hydrocephalus (NPH)—a treatable cause of dementia—if accompanied by urinary incontinence and cognitive decline.*

Musculoskeletal system

- Check gait and balance by observing the patient walk from the waiting room to the office. Look for reliance on furniture or other objects for support during ambulation.
- Note whether the patient uses assistive devices such as a cane, walker, or wheelchair, and assess their effectiveness and proper use.

Laboratory and Diagnostic Testing

Basic laboratory tests

Consider these essential screening tests for most older adults with psychiatric symptoms:

- *Complete blood count:* Identifies anemia or infections that may underlie psychiatric symptoms, such as depression, anxiety, or cognitive impairment.
- *Thyroid function tests:* Hyperthyroidism can present with symptoms of anxiety, agitation, and mood instability, while hypothyroidism is associated with depression and lethargy.
- *Electrolyte panel:* Imbalances such as in hyponatremia or hypercalcemia can cause confusion, mood changes, and, in severe cases, delirium.
- *Vitamin B12 and folate levels:* Deficiencies may lead to depression, cognitive decline, and other neurological changes.
- *Liver and kidney function tests:* Impaired function results in a buildup of toxins, like ammonia or urea, which can cause symptoms ranging from subtle cognitive impairment to overt encephalopathy.
- *Fasting glucose and HbA1c:* Diabetes and fluctuating blood sugar levels can affect mood and contribute to anxiety and cognitive changes. Antipsychotics increase the risk for metabolic syndrome, which in turn is associated with hyperglycemia.
- *Lipid panel:* Antipsychotics can cause metabolic syndrome, which is also linked with hyperlipidemia. Monitor lipids before and during treatment with antipsychotics.
- *Urinalysis:* Urinary tract infections often lead to acute confusion or delirium in older patients.
- *Toxicology screening:* Important for detecting substance use that can cause or exacerbate psychiatric conditions, including depression, anxiety, and psychosis.
- *Vitamin D levels:* Deficiency is associated with an increased risk of depression and cognitive decline.

- *Electrocardiogram (ECG)*
  - Cardiac diseases (eg, arrhythmias) can trigger anxiety or panic attacks as a result of physical symptoms like palpitations or tachycardia.
  - Older adults are at higher risk for developing QTc prolongation with antipsychotics, tricyclic antidepressants, and citalopram.

Advanced diagnostic tools

Many of these tests are typically interpreted by specialists, but understanding their role helps us coordinate care effectively:

- *Neuropsychological testing:* Administered by neuropsychologists, neuropsychological testing is the gold standard for diagnosing dementia. Think of neuropsychological testing as a detailed map of cognitive function. While basic screening tells us something is wrong, neuropsychological testing tells us:
  - Which specific cognitive domains are affected.
  - Whether the pattern suggests Alzheimer's dementia (AD), frontotemporal dementia (FTD), or another condition.
  - If symptoms are more likely due to depression or another mental illness, rather than dementia.
- *Brain imaging (CT/MRI):* Useful for diagnosing nonpsychiatric conditions that impact mental status, such as strokes, tumors, and normal pressure hydrocephalus, as well as for detecting structural brain changes associated with dementia.
  - Key uses
    - Evaluating new-onset psychiatric symptoms after 65.
    - Assessing unexplained personality changes.
    - Investigating cognitive decline.
- *Positron emission tomography (PET) scan:* A PET scan reveals brain activity patterns.
  - Key uses
    - Useful when you are stuck between different diagnoses (like AD vs FTD vs another neurodegenerative disease)
    - Recently, insurances have been approving more PET scans, especially to help distinguish AD from FTD or before starting an anti-amyloid therapy for AD.
- *Lumbar puncture (LP)*
  - Key uses
    - Dementia diagnosis
      - Measures specific proteins (tau and beta-amyloid) that can confirm AD with high accuracy.
      - Can identify rare but serious causes of dementia like Creutzfeldt-Jakob Disease (CJD).
    - Evaluate for unexplained altered mental status (AMS).
    - Infection detection
      - Rules out brain infections that can masquerade as psychiatric illness.
      - Can identify infections that blood tests might miss.
- *Genetic testing*
  - Early-onset AD
    - Key genes: APP, PSEN1, and PSEN2.
    - Consider when dementia starts before age 65.
    - Especially important when there is a strong family history.
  - Treatment planning for AD
    - APOE ε4 testing helps predict risk of side effects with anti-amyloid therapy
    - APOE ε4 is not used to predict who will develop AD.
  - FTD
    - Look for MAPT, GRN, and C9orf72 mutations.
    - Most valuable when multiple family members have FTD.
    - Can help confirm diagnosis in unclear cases.
  - Genetic testing should be accompanied by genetic counseling. A positive test has implications not only for the patient but also for their descendants.
- *Sleep study*
  - A sleep study is essential to diagnose sleep apnea, which may lead to daytime fatigue, cognitive impairment, and mood disturbances. Sleep apnea can also cause strokes, further impacting cognition.
  - Other sleep disorders such as restless legs syndrome, rapid eye movement sleep behavior disorder, and periodic limb movement disorder may be detected via a sleep study. They too contribute to poor sleep, daytime fatigue, and mood disturbances.

CLINICAL PEARL: *Always consider sleep apnea in an older adult presenting with new or worsening daytime fatigue, difficulty concentrating, and cognitive decline.*

Medical Mimics in Geriatric Psychiatry

Medical mimics refer to medical conditions that can present with psychiatric symptoms. These conditions, if misdiagnosed as primary psychiatric disorders, lead to inappropriate treatment and worsened outcomes. While there are many possible medical mimics, I will focus on conditions that commonly perplex us in geriatric psychiatry.

Autoimmune Disorders

Systemic Lupus Erythematosus (SLE)

A chronic condition impacting multiple systems that begins in adulthood and continues into later life.

- *Symptoms*
  - Typical symptoms: Fever, joint pain, rash, and kidney involvement.
  - Neuropsychiatric symptoms (NPS) in later life: Mood/anxiety disorders and cognitive dysfunction that results in memory impairment, difficulty concentrating, and executive dysfunction.
  - Patients can occasionally have psychosis manifesting as paranoia or hallucinations.
- *Laboratory tests:* Antinuclear antibody (ANA), anti-dsDNA, complement levels.
- *Management*
  - If symptoms occur during an exacerbation, coordinate care with the patient's rheumatologist, since some symptoms can also be side effects of SLE treatment (eg, psychosis from high-dose corticosteroids).
  - *Neuropsychiatric symptoms*
    - Cognitive dysfunction/dementia
      - Pharmacologic treatment: Cognitive enhancers (eg, donepezil, memantine) may be considered.
    - Mood and anxiety disorders
      - Pharmacologic treatment: Antidepressants (eg, selective serotonin reuptake inhibitors [SSRIs], serotonin-norepinephrine reuptake inhibitors [SNRIs]), anxiolytics, mood stabilizers (eg, lithium, valproate).
      - Nonpharmacologic treatment: Cognitive behavioral therapy (CBT), supportive therapy.
    - Psychosis
      - Pharmacologic treatment: Second-generation antipsychotics (eg, risperidone, olanzapine).

Anti-N-Methyl-D-Aspartate receptor encephalitis (anti-NMDAR encephalitis)

- Relatively rare and more commonly associated with younger women, but it can occur in older adults. It is critical to recognize it early, so that treatment delays do not occur.
  - *Neuropsychiatric symptoms*
    - 95% of older adults with anti-NMDAR encephalitis will have behavioral and cognitive symptoms, therefore, they may present first in mental health settings. Consider the diagnosis when:
      - The person has no prior history of psychiatric disturbances.
      - The patient exhibits atypical psychosis, sudden onset, and has a fluctuating pattern of delusions.
      - There are signs of akinetic or hyperkinetic mobility disturbances, including catatonia.
      - Seizures are a prominent part of the history; they complicate 40% of cases (Gine-Serven E et al, *Gen Hosp Psychiatry* 2022:74:71-77).
  - *Tests:* cerebrospinal fluid analysis—anti-NMDAR antibodies, EEG, brain MRI.
- Management
  - *Immunotherapy:* First-line treatment includes steroids, intravenous immunoglobulin, or plasmapheresis.
  - *NPS:* Avoid benzodiazepines and antipsychotics.
    - Benzodiazepines can worsen respiratory depression and confusion.
    - There may be an association between antipsychotics and neuroleptic malignant syndrome in people with anti-NMDAR encephalitis.
    - Balance the risk of psychotropic medications against the potential benefit of decreasing NPS symptoms and dangerous behaviors.
    - Anticonvulsants like divalproex or gabapentin may be reasonable first-step options (Beattie M et al, *BJPsych Bull* 2021;46(4):1-7).

Hypothyroidism

A condition in which the thyroid gland doesn't produce enough thyroid hormone. It becomes more common with age. In older adults, the presentation of hypothyroidism can be subtle and mistaken for other conditions related to aging.

Symptoms

- *General:* Fatigue, weight gain, cold intolerance, dry skin and hair, constipation, muscle weakness.
- *Neuropsychiatric symptoms*
  - Apathy: Lack of interest or motivation.

- Cognitive impairment/dementia: Deficits in memory, psychomotor slowing, and impaired visuospatial skills (none of which show consistent recovery with thyroid treatment) (Dugbartey AT, *Arch Intern Med* 1998;158(13):1413–1418).
- Depression: Low mood, lack of interest in activities, and feelings of hopelessness.
- Psychosis (myxedema madness): Delusions and hallucinations can emerge after the onset of physical symptoms, often after an untreated period of years or months. Myxedema madness most often occurs in older women (Ueno S et al, *J Med Case Rep* 2015;9:264).

Thyroid function tests

- *Thyroid-stimulating hormone (TSH):* Elevated levels indicate hypothyroidism.
- *Free T4 (thyroxine):* Low levels confirm the diagnosis.
- *Anti-thyroid antibodies:* Detect autoimmune thyroid disorders (eg, Hashimoto's thyroiditis).

Management

- *Primary treatment:* Address the underlying hypothyroidism, though many patients will require additional treatment for NPS.
- *Neuropsychiatric symptoms*
  - Cognitive impairment/dementia: Dementia due to hypothyroidism is likely not fully reversible even with thyroid treatment. Consider acetylcholinesterase Inhibitors (eg, donepezil, rivastigmine) if cognitive impairment is significant.
  - Depression: SSRIs, SNRIs, and CBT.
  - Psychosis: Second-generation antipsychotics (eg, risperidone, olanzapine) are preferred due to their better side effect profiles.

PRACTICE POINT: *Check thyroid function even when patients are already on thyroid replacement. Older adults' thyroid needs change over time, and both over- and under-replacement can cause psychiatric symptoms.*

Neurological

Stroke or cerebrovascular accident (CVA)

- Occurs when the blood supply to a part of the brain is interrupted, causing neuronal cell death.
  - Ischemic: Resulting from blockage or narrowing of brain arteries.
  - Hemorrhagic: When a blood vessel in the brain bursts, causing bleeding in or around the brain.

Neuropsychiatric symptoms

- *Anxiety:* Found in 25% of people following a stroke; often comorbid with depression, fatigue, and poor social support.
- *Apathy:* Manifests as a lack of motivation, loss of initiative, decreased goal-directed activity, and emotional blunting. Prevalence is about 40%. It can start acutely or develop chronically. Patients with post-stroke apathy have greater cognitive impairment (https://tinyurl.com/2n49vsub).
- *Depression:* Post-stroke depression (PSD) occurs in about 30% of stroke patients, with onset ranging from immediately after the stroke to months later. It is not always correlated with stroke-related disability.

Management

- *Anxiety:* SSRIs (eg, sertraline, escitalopram) are first-line choices along with psychotherapy.
- *Apathy:* Psychostimulants (eg, methylphenidate, modafinil) and bupropion may be helpful for treating post-stroke apathy. However, avoid bupropion in patients at risk for seizures, especially those who have experienced a hemorrhagic stroke. Non-pharmacological strategies such as structured routines, behavioral activation, and problem-solving therapy may also be of benefit.
- *PSD*
  - Antidepressants: SSRIs/SNRIs such as fluoxetine, duloxetine, and escitalopram are commonly used and may even improve motor recovery. However, they may slightly increase bleeding risk, especially in patients taking anticoagulants. Although this risk appears to be low overall, clinicians should exercise caution. Mirtazapine is a suitable alternative with lower bleeding risk.
  - Psychotherapy: CBT and psychoeducation have demonstrated effectiveness for PSD. Integrating psychotherapy with pharmacological treatment often yields the best outcomes (Starkstein SE and Hayhow BD, *Curr Treat Options Neurol* 2019;21(7):31).

Wernicke/Korsakoff Syndrome

Wernicke/Korsakoff Syndrome (WKS) is a spectrum of disorders, ranging from Wernicke's Encephalopathy (WE), which is reversible, to Korsakoff Syndrome (KS), which is irreversible and develops if WE is not treated promptly. WKS is caused by thiamine deficiency. In older adults, this may be related to alcohol use disorder (AUD) or malnutrition from other sources, including GI diseases or food insecurity.

Symptoms

- *WE*
  - Ophthalmoplegia: Difficulty looking to the side from lateral rectus nerve palsy. It may present as blurred vision or difficulty tracking objects.
  - Ataxia: Wide-based, short-stepped gait with difficulty standing or walking. Ask about a history of falls and also consider a secondary subdural hemorrhage.
  - Confusion: Disorientation, memory impairment, decreased consciousness, or apathy with acute or subacute onset. Mentation is often fluctuating.
- *KS*
  - Confabulation: People with KS will make up stories without the intention to deceive. These false memories can be subtle to elaborate and detailed.
  - Cognitive impairment/dementia: Inability to form new memories.
  - Hallucinations

Tests

Only about 20% of patients with WE will exhibit all three signs. Do not over-rely on tests such as thiamine levels and brain MRIs, as they too are often unremarkable (Isenberg-Grzeda E et al, *Psychosomatics* 2012;53(6):507–516).

PRACTICE POINT: *Always administer thiamine before glucose to avoid exacerbating symptoms. Glucose can precipitate KS or worsen WE in thiamine-deficient patients.*

Management

- Since the full triad rarely presents, it is advisable to begin treatment in the presence of one or two signs, especially if the patient has risk factors for WE.
- *WE*
  - Thiamine replacement: The current practice is to administer high-dose thiamine intravenously. Thiamine is a water-soluble vitamin, so any excess will be excreted, preventing toxic buildup. IV or IM thiamine is preferred initially as many patients with AUD or other GI disturbances poorly absorb oral thiamine.

Table 2: **Thiamine for Wernicke/Korsakoff Syndrome**

Medication	Dosage	Notes
Intravenous Thiamine	500 mg IV three times daily	For two to three days, then 250 mg daily for five days
Oral Thiamine	100 mg BID	After initial IV treatment

(Isenberg-Grzeda E et al 2012)

- *KS*
  - Thiamine replacement: Although KS is irreversible, occasionally patients will have some recovery from high-dose IV thiamine.
  - Disposition: Depending upon the degree of impairment in cognition and activities of daily living, patients may need residential care.

Subdural Hemorrhage (SDH)

SDH is a type of intracranial bleeding that occurs between the dura mater and the arachnoid mater. It can be acute, subacute, or chronic. Older adults are at higher risk for developing SDH following trauma than younger people. Risk factors are recent falls, head trauma, anticoagulant use, alcohol use, and history of coagulopathy.

Neuropsychiatric symptoms

- *General:* Drowsiness, altered level of consciousness, dizziness, nausea.
- *Cognitive impairment:* Memory problems, confusion, slowed thinking, executive dysfunction. Memory loss may be gradual in people with chronic SDH, making it easy to confuse with dementia.
- *Behavioral changes:* Personality changes, irritability, apathy, agitation. SDH can be mistaken for a primary psychiatric disorder such as depression or bipolar disorder.
- *Mood and anxiety disorders:* New-onset depression, anxiety, mood swings. These symptoms can develop as the hematoma exerts pressure on brain tissue.

Tests

Head CT: First-line choice to detect acute or chronic subdural hematoma.

Management

- Referral to the emergency department, neurology, or neurosurgery
- Cognitive impairment and behavioral changes
  - Medications: Consider cholinesterase inhibitors (eg, donepezil, rivastigmine) if there is a significant cognitive component or if memory loss does not improve after medical management.
  - Nonpharmacologic: Cognitive rehabilitation.
- Mood disorders

- Antidepressants: SSRIs (eg, sertraline, escitalopram) or SNRIs (eg, venlafaxine, duloxetine) can be used to treat depression and anxiety, though, they may increase bleeding risk. Mirtazapine is an alternative with lower risk.
- Mood stabilizers: For mood swings/irritability, consider mood stabilizers (lithium, lamotrigine).

CLINICAL PEARL: A *chronic subdural hemorrhage can mimic dementia or depression but is reversible with prompt recognition and treatment. A noncontrast CT scan of the head is the diagnostic study of choice.*

Neuroimaging in Late-Life Psychiatric Conditions

Advanced imaging modalities, including magnetic resonance imaging (MRI), computed tomography (CT), positron emission tomography (PET), and single photon emission computed tomography (SPECT), aid in accurate diagnosis, treatment planning, and monitoring of late-life psychiatric disorders such as dementia. This fact sheet highlights applications of imaging, focusing on specific findings and their clinical implications.

CASE VIGNETTE: *Ms. Clarke, a 75-year-old woman, presents with short-term memory loss and several episodes of getting lost while walking in her neighborhood. MRI shows medial temporal lobe atrophy. Amyloid PET is positive for amyloid plaques. She is diagnosed with major neurocognitive disorder due to probable Alzheimer's disease, mild. Ms. Clarke is started on an anti-amyloid medication, lecanemab (Leqembi). The patient is also referred to a senior center for socialization and cognitive stimulation.*

Types of Imaging in Late-Life Psychiatry

- *CT:* Widely available, faster, and less expensive than an MRI but provides less detailed images. Used to rule out structural brain abnormalities, such as tumors, or when results are needed rapidly to evaluate for a stroke or brain hemorrhage.
- *MRI:* Detects anatomical changes in brain structures. It is used in diagnosing neurodegenerative diseases such as Alzheimer's dementia (AD) and vascular dementia (VaD).
- *PET:* Fluorodeoxyglucose (FDG)-PET measures glucose metabolism in the brain. Glucose is the brain's main fuel, so areas of hypometabolism indicate areas with reduced activity. This can help distinguish between different types of dementia.
  - Amyloid PET detects amyloid plaques in the brain, an important feature of AD.
  - Tau PET finds abnormal tau deposits in the brain, which also occur in AD. The buildup of phosphorylated tau correlates with cognitive and functional decline in people with AD.
- *SPECT:* Provides information on cerebral blood flow and is used in evaluating conditions like dementia. It is less expensive than a PET scan but also less detailed.

When to Order Imaging?

Dementia evaluation

- *Initial evaluation:* Order a brain MRI or, if an MRI is contraindicated (due to claustrophobia or an implanted device not compatible with an MRI, like an older pacemaker), order a head CT.
- *Rapid cognitive decline:* Order imaging if there is a sudden or rapid decline in cognitive function to rule out acute conditions like a subarachnoid hemorrhage or stroke. Consider referring the patient to a neurologist or the emergency department, depending on the acuity of the situation.

New-onset psychiatric disorder

Except for dementia and delirium, most psychiatric disorders manifest earlier in life. Therefore, any new-onset psychiatric disorder (eg, a patient experiencing a major depressive episode for the first time at age 70) in an older adult should be presumed to be secondary to an underlying medical condition until proven otherwise. In these situations, consider ordering a head CT or brain MRI as part of your workup.

Application of Imaging in Specific Psychiatric Conditions

AD and other dementias

While neuroimaging cannot definitively diagnose dementia, it can provide valuable information to support a diagnosis or help distinguish among different types of dementia. PET and SPECT scans can detect early changes in brain activity, often before structural changes like atrophy become apparent on MRI or CT scans

- *Structural MRI*
  - Atrophy
    - The pattern of brain atrophy can provide valuable clues about the underlying type of dementia. In AD, atrophy typically affects the medial temporal lobe, leading to impairments in short-term memory. In contrast, frontotemporal dementia (FTD) is characterized by atrophy of the frontal and temporal lobes (hence the name), resulting in deficits in behavior, language, and personality.
  - Vascular contributions
    - White matter hyperintensities (WMH) are abnormalities in white matter that appear as bright spots on T2-weighted MRI images. They are often linked to cerebrovascular risk factors such as hypertension and smoking. WMH can disrupt communication between brain regions and have been associated with a variety of

cognitive and neuropsychiatric disorders, including late-life depression, bipolar disorder, and vascular dementia. See *The Carlat Geriatric Psychiatry Report,* July/August/September 2022.

- *FDG-PET*
  - AD: Characteristic patterns of hypometabolism are observed in the bilateral parietal and temporal lobes, posterior cingulate, and cuneus regions.
  - FTD: Hypometabolism is predominantly found in the frontal and temporal lobes, typically asymmetrical and often more pronounced on the right side.

PRACTICE POINT: *The distinct patterns of hypometabolism seen in AD and FTD make FDG-PET a valuable tool for differentiating between these conditions. Medicare covers FDG-PET scans for patients who meet diagnostic criteria for both AD and FTD, aiding in the differential.*

  - Dementia with Lewy bodies (DLB): Posterior parietal and occipital lobe hypometabolism is found in DLB, correlating with visual hallucinations and visuospatial disturbances.
- *Amyloid PET*
  - Identifies amyloid plaques, which aids in the diagnosis of AD. Amyloid deposition is necessary for AD diagnosis but also occurs in other conditions like traumatic brain injury or even in normal aging. A negative scan excludes AD.
  - Amyloid PET establishes the presence of beta-amyloid pathology, making patients with AD potentially eligible for one of the anti-amyloid treatments.
- *Tau PET*
  - Detects tau protein tangles, which correlate with neurodegeneration and cognitive decline in AD.

Table 3: **Imaging Findings in Different Types of Dementia**

Dementia Type	Imaging Modality	Key Findings
Alzheimer's Dementia	MRI	Medial temporal lobe atrophy
	FDG-PET	Hypometabolism in bilateral temporal and parietal lobes and in the posterior cingulate
	Amyloid PET	Positive for amyloid plaques
	Tau PET	Positive for tau deposition
Frontotemporal Dementia	MRI	Atrophy in anterior frontal and temporal lobes
	FDG-PET	Hypometabolism in anterior frontal and temporal lobes, often asymmetrical
Lewy Body Dementia	FDG-PET	Hypometabolism in posterior parietal and occipital lobes
Vascular Dementia	MRI	Extensive WMH, infarcts

Source: Shivamurthy VKN et al, *AJR Am J Roentgrenol* 2015;204(1):W76-W85.

Late-life mood disorders

- *MRI*
  - White matter hyperintensities: Increased WMH are commonly seen in late-life depression and especially in people with older-age bipolar disorder.
  - Hippocampal atrophy: Associated with depression complicated by cognitive deficits. It is reversible with antidepressant treatment, but late-life depression is either an early sign of dementia or increases the risk of dementia. Accordingly, patients with late-life depression should be monitored closely for the emergence of cognitive impairment.

COMMON LATE-LIFE PSYCHIATRIC DISORDERS

Anxiety Disorders

Anxiety in the Older Adult

Anxiety disorders occur in 8% of older adults and are more common than late-life mood disorders, yet they are often underdiagnosed and undertreated (Aggarwal R et al, *Focus* 2017;15(2):157–161).

CASE VIGNETTE: *Mrs. Chen, 82, presents with stomach problems and withdrawal from activities. While denying anxiety, she shows constant health worries, frequent medical appointments, and repeated calls to her children "to make sure they're okay." Diagnosed with generalized anxiety disorder (GAD), she improves with sertraline 50 mg daily and deep breathing techniques, resuming her social activities after eight weeks.*

Recognizing Anxiety in Older Adults

Verbal cues

- *Expressions of worry or fear*
  - Listen for repeated expressions of worry about health, safety, finances, or family. Older adults might express concerns about becoming a burden or express fear of future events.
- *Change in language*
  - Note any increase in conversations about feeling overwhelmed, stressed, or unable to cope with daily routines or changing circumstances.
  - Older adults may describe anxiety differently than younger people, using terms like "nervousness" or "worry" rather than "anxiety" (Lutz J et al, *Med Clin North Am* 2020;104(5):843-854).

Complaints of physical symptoms

- Pay attention to complaints that might be due to underlying anxiety, such as unexplained aches, increased fatigue, headaches, or gastrointestinal issues without a clear medical cause.
- Physical symptoms of anxiety (eg, heart palpitations, dizziness) may be misattributed to medical conditions, leading to under recognition of anxiety.

Behavioral signs

- *Avoidance behavior:* Observe if the individual starts to avoid social interactions, activities they once enjoyed, or specific situations, like going outside or attending appointments.
- *Changes in sleep patterns:* Difficulty falling asleep, staying asleep, or excessive sleep can be signs of anxiety. Older adults might mention having racing thoughts at night or fearing the dark.
- *Increased irritability or restlessness:* Older adults with anxiety may exhibit restlessness, have difficulty sitting still, or become more easily irritated by minor issues.

Physical symptoms/reactions

Look for signs of restlessness, trembling, muscle tension, or being easily startled. Some older adults have physical reactions to anxiety, such as sweating, rapid heartbeat, or breathing difficulties.

Common Late-Life Anxiety Disorders

GAD

- Ask: "Are you a worrier?"
- GAD is characterized by excessive, uncontrollable worry about different topics.
- Older adults have a greater variety of worry topics than younger adults, including memory loss, medical illnesses, finances, and safety. They worry less about the future and work.
- Late-onset GAD is challenging to distinguish from everyday aging concerns, but the worries are life-impairing, persistent, and disproportionate to the situation in people with GAD.
- Of the anxiety disorders, GAD and agoraphobia (avoidance of situations where escape may be difficult or help not available) are the most likely to start in old age (Canuto A et al, *Am J Geriatr Psychiatry* 2018;26(2):174-185).

Specific phobias

- Ask: "Do you have any specific fears?"
- High prevalence in older adults, often related to fears of falling, injury, or medical procedures.
- These phobias can significantly restrict activities and contribute to functional decline.

Panic disorder (PD)

- Ask: "Do you get panic attacks?"

- Most cases in older adults represent a continuation of earlier-life PD or are associated with cardiopulmonary disease, eg, COPD.
- Physical symptoms and avoidance behaviors may be less intense compared to younger adults.

Social anxiety disorder (SAD)

- Ask: "Are you uncomfortable in social situations?"
- Older people experience less SAD than their younger counterparts (Pary R et al, *Prim Care Companion CNS Disord* 2019;21(1):18nr02335).
- SAD is more common in older adults who report stressful life events, such as the death of a spouse, depression, or phobias.

Specific Later-Life Anxiety Syndromes

Fear of falling

- Ask: "Have you experienced previous falls or near falls?" and "Do you practice any specific behaviors to avoid falls?"
- A significant proportion of older adults experience fear of falling, which can lead to avoidance of activities, social withdrawal, reduced physical fitness, and, paradoxically, an increased risk of falls.
- In severe cases, the fear of falling can even lead to trepidation about leaving the house.
- Fear of falling necessitates interventions ranging from physical therapy to address mobility and balance, to psychological interventions aimed at reducing fear and anxiety.

Hoarding disorder

- Ask: "Do you have difficulty discarding or parting with possessions, regardless of their value?"
- This condition leads to cluttered living spaces, which can impair daily functioning and pose significant safety risks, such as falls, fires, and infestation.
- Hoarding is particularly challenging in older adults due to extended accumulation periods and resistance to intervention.
- Address underlying anxiety, offer support, and involve family or community resources to help discard possessions, with the patient's permission.

Anxiety as a prodrome of cognitive impairment

- Anxiety in older adults can be an early indicator of cognitive decline or a prodromal symptom of a major neurocognitive disorder, such as Alzheimer's dementia.
- Monitor older adults with new-onset anxiety for cognitive changes.
- Cognitive assessments can help to differentiate between primary anxiety disorders and anxiety secondary to cognitive impairment.

Choosing Anxiolytics for Older Adults

This fact sheet focuses on the pharmacological management of anxiety disorders in older adults, highlighting key considerations for dosages, drug selection, and monitoring to ensure safety and efficacy.

Strategy for Choosing Anxiolytics in Older Adults

Stepwise approach: Use a structured strategy to guide medication choice based on patient-specific factors. See "Table 4: Anxiolytics for Late-Life Anxiety Disorders."

- Start with selective serotonin reuptake inhibitors (SSRIs) for broad-spectrum efficacy and a safer side effect profile. Consider sertraline or escitalopram as your first-line options.
- Progress to serotonin-norepinephrine reuptake inhibitors (SNRIs) like venlafaxine or duloxetine if SSRIs are ineffective, particularly in patients with comorbid chronic pain.
- For adjunctive treatment or intolerance to second-line agents, consider buspirone or gabapentin/pregabalin.
- Reserve benzodiazepines or antipsychotics for severe, refractory cases or acute exacerbations, with close monitoring.

PRACTICE POINT: *Start at the lowest possible dose and titrate every 2–4 weeks based on response and tolerability. Allow at least 8–12 weeks at a therapeutic dose before assessing efficacy. Anxiety disorders often respond more slowly to medications in older adults than in younger populations.*

Table 4: **Anxiolytics for Late-Life Anxiety Disorders**

Class/Category	Medication/ Intervention	Dosage	Considerations
Selective Serotonin Reuptake Inhibitors (SSRIs) • SSRIs are effective for a range of late-life anxiety disorders, including generalized anxiety disorder (GAD), panic disorder, and social anxiety disorder. • SSRIs have the safest side effect profile compared to other classes.	Citalopram	Start at 10 mg daily; titrate to maximum dose of 20 mg daily	Similar considerations as escitalopram Black box warning for QTc prolongation at doses >20 mg/day due to risk of sudden cardiac death
	Escitalopram	Start at 5 mg daily; titrate to 10-20 mg daily	Monitor for hyponatremia, GI issues, sexual dysfunction, and less commonly, falls, fractures, and bleeding
	Fluoxetine	Avoid if possible	Similar considerations as escitalopram. Potent CYP2D6 inhibitor; high potential for drug-drug interactions
	Paroxetine	Avoid if possible	Similar considerations as escitalopram. Significant anticholinergic activity and CYP2D6 inhibition
	Sertraline	Start at 25 mg daily; titrate to 50–200 mg daily	Similar considerations as escitalopram. Higher rate of GI side effects than other SSRIs.
Serotonin-Norepinephrine Reuptake Inhibitors (SNRIs) • Effective for GAD	Desvenlafaxine	Start at 25 mg daily; maintenance dose is 50 mg daily	Active metabolite of venlafaxine Requires renal dose adjustment
	Duloxetine	Start at 30 mg daily; therapeutic range 60–90 mg daily	Helpful for comorbid chronic pain or neuropathic pain Monitor blood pressure and watch for hyponatremia, sexual dysfunction, GI side effects, and less commonly, falls, fractures, and bleeding Monitor LFTs every 6 months for hepatoxicity (rare) Watch for urinary retention which can contribute to UTIs
	Venlafaxine XR	Start at 37.5 mg daily; titrate to 75–225 mg daily	Monitor blood pressure and watch for hyponatremia, sexual dysfunction, and GI side effects and less commonly, falls, fractures, and bleeding
Buspirone • An option for GAD	Buspirone	Start at 7.5 mg twice daily; titrate to 10–45 mg/day divided into 2–3 doses	Effective for cognitive symptoms of anxiety Well tolerated with less risk of dependency Onset of action is delayed by several weeks
Gabapentinoids • Consider for GAD or social anxiety	Gabapentin	300–1200 mg daily, divided into 3 doses	Helps with comorbid neuropathic pain Adjust dose for renal impairment Can be prescribed as monotherapy or as an adjunct to SSRIs/SNRIs. Monitor for dizziness, fatigue, edema May cause drowsiness, leading to falls and injury, as well as have additive sedative effects when combined with other CNS depressants
	Pregabalin	Start at 25 mg twice daily; titrate to 150–450 mg per day, divided into 2–3 doses	Similar to gabapentin

(table continues)

Table 4: **Anxiolytics for Late-Life Anxiety Disorders** *(continued)*

Class/Category	Medication/ Intervention	Dosage	Considerations
Benzodiazepines • Helpful for severe GAD or panic attacks	Lorazepam	0.5–1 mg as needed	Short-term or acute use only Monitor for cognitive impairment, dependence, and falls Preferred for older adults due to shorter half-life and few active metabolites
	Oxazepam	10–15 mg as needed	Same as lorazepam Delayed onset of action
Beta-blockers • An option for situational and performance anxiety	Propranolol	10–40 mg about 1 hour before event	Monitor for hypotension and bradycardia Avoid prescribing for patients with cardiovascular conditions or those who are taking antihypertensive or antiarrhythmic agents
Antipsychotics	Quetiapine	25–50 mg at bedtime	Reserved for severe anxiety unresponsive to other treatments Monitor for metabolic syndrome, extrapyramidal symptoms, and tardive dyskinesia
Alternative Therapies	Lavender oil (Silexan)	80 mg once daily; up to 160 mg in some studies	Comparable to low-dose lorazepam (Yap WS et al, Sci Rep 2019;9(1):18042) Well-tolerated with mild GI side effects including "lavender burps" Nonsedating and nonhabit-forming
	Saffron extract	20–30 mg daily	Potential efficacy for mild to moderate anxiety Anti-inflammatory and antioxidant properties Watch for appetite changes and drowsiness

Benzodiazepines in Older Adults

The percentage of people who use benzodiazepines (BZD) increases with age, reaching 9% in those 65 to 80. The proportion of chronic BZD use also rises with age, peaking at 32% in this age group. Psychiatrists account for 6% of BZD prescriptions in older adults (Olfson M et al, *JAMA Psychiatry* 2015;72(2):136-142). Benzodiazepines are commonly prescribed because of their perceived effectiveness and rapid onset of action. They offer quick relief, unlike antidepressants, which require four to six weeks to take effect. However, BZDs have significant risks in older adults and are a last-resort choice for most conditions. This fact sheet will provide an overview for clinicians on BZD use in older adults.

Table 5: **Commonly Prescribed Benzodiazepines in Older Adults**

Type	Benzodiazepine	Half-life (hours)	Potency	FDA-Approved Diagnoses	Lorazepam Equivalents (mg)
Short-acting	Lorazepam (Ativan)	10–20	High	Anxiety, insomnia, seizures, premedication for procedures	1
	Oxazepam (Serax)	5–15	Low	Anxiety, alcohol withdrawal	15
Intermediate-acting	Alprazolam (Xanax)	6–20	High	Anxiety, panic disorder	0.5
	Temazepam (Restoril)	8–22	Low	Insomnia	30
Long-acting	Chlordiazepoxide (Librium)	5–30	Low	Anxiety, alcohol withdrawal	25
	Clonazepam (Klonopin)	30–40	High	Panic disorder, seizures	0.5
	Diazepam (Valium)	20–50	Low	Anxiety, muscle spasms, seizures, alcohol withdrawal	5

Source: Singh S and Sarkar S, *Journal of Geriatric Mental Health* 2016;3(2):123-130.

Indications for Use

Anxiety disorders

Evidence shows the best use for BZDs in older adults is for generalized anxiety disorder. BZDs may be considered when other treatments have failed or if rapid symptomatic relief is needed.

- *Alprazolam:* Helpful in a pinch for someone who might use it rarely for a panic attack. Can lead to a severe withdrawal syndrome, including withdrawal seizures, and has high abuse potential. Frequent use can also lessen the benefit of psychotherapy.
- *Clonazepam and diazepam:* Avoid in older adults due to longer half-lives, increased fall risk, and tendency to build up metabolites.
- *Lorazepam*: 0.5–2 mg at HS or divided twice daily. It is the preferred choice as it does not linger in the system due to its shorter half-life. It also does not build up metabolites, which can lead to excess sedation and falls. Lorazepam has a lower risk of abuse.
- *Oxazepam:* 10 mg daily to 15 mg TID. Lower abuse potential, but some patients find it does not have a potent antianxiety effect, at least compared to the others. It also takes more than one hour to work.

Insomnia

Use cautiously for the short-term management of severe insomnia after other treatments have failed.

- Lorazepam: 0.5–1 mg at bedtime.
- Temazepam: 7.5–15 mg at bedtime.

REM behavior disorder (RBD)

RBD can result in violent movements and vocalizations while dreaming; it may predict the onset of Parkinson's disease (PD).

- *Clonazepam:* 0.25–2 mg at bedtime, with most people maintained at 1 mg qHS.
- Other options:
  - Melatonin: 3–12 mg at bedtime.
  - Pramipexole: 0.125–0.5 mg at bedtime.
  - Transdermal rivastigmine: 4.6–13.3 mg; consider for patients with comorbid mild cognitive impairment or PD dementia.

Alcohol withdrawal

- Clinical Institute Withdrawal Assessment (CIWA) protocols utilizing BZDs remain the recommended strategy for detoxing older adults from alcohol.
- Because of concerns for accumulation, lorazepam and oxazepam are the recommended detoxing agents over diazepam or chlordiazepoxide.

Acute agitation

- For most situations, an atypical or typical antipsychotic will be the first-line intervention.
- If the antipsychotic is not effective or if the patient has PD or dementia with Lewy bodies (DLB), then utilize a low-dose benzodiazepine (eg, lorazepam 0.5–1mg IM or IV). Avoid high-potency antipsychotics (eg, olanzapine or haloperidol) in patients with PD/DLB.

Risks and Adverse Effects

Cognitive impairment

- Increased risk of memory impairment, delirium, and possibly dementia.
- Studies show that impaired visuospatial ability, processing speed, and verbal learning occurs with long-term BZD use. Although cognition can improve after BZDs are withdrawn, patients do not return to baseline. The overall impact of the impairment appears to be minor, though (Stewart SA, *J Clin Psychiatry* 2005;66 Suppl 2:9-13).

Dependence

- The risk of dependence may be lower than previously thought. Still, in those with a history of substance abuse or for those over age 80, there remains a significantly higher chance of prolonged use and dose escalation (Rosenqvist TW et al, *Am J Psychiatry* 2024;181(3):246-254).
- For all older adults, the main reasons for caution are cognitive issues, falls, and drug interactions.

Falls and fractures

- 50% increased risk of falls due to sedation, dizziness, and impaired coordination.
- BZDs are an independent risk factor for falls in older adults (Bakken MS et al, *Eur J Clin Pharmacol* 2014;70(7):873–880).
- Falls can lead to fractures, particularly concerning are hip fractures, which have substantial morbidity and mortality.

Interactions with other substances

Dangerous BZD interactions occur when they are combined with alcohol, opioids, gabapentinoids, and other sedative-hypnotics. These combinations carry an increased risk of sedation, falls, and respiratory depression.

Motor vehicle accidents (MVAs)

- Older adults are already at higher risk for MVAs due to reduced coordination, visual changes, slowed processing speed, polypharmacy, and other factors.
- BZDs approximately double the risk of an MVA. The risk for older drivers is higher when they take longer-acting and larger quantities of BZDs (Thomas RE, *Can Fam Physician* 1998;44:799-808).

Respiratory depression

- BZDs increase the risk of difficulty breathing, especially in patients with underlying respiratory conditions such as chronic obstructive pulmonary disease or sleep apnea.
- They should be prescribed cautiously and closely monitored in patients with respiratory conditions.

Dosing Considerations

Start low, go slow

- Initiate treatment with the lowest effective dose.
- Gradually increase the dose, while monitoring for efficacy and adverse effects.

Short-term use

- Aim for the shortest duration of use to minimize risks.
- Regularly reassess the need for continued BZD therapy.
- Shorter half-life BZDs are preferred over longer half-life ones.

Dose titration and discontinuation of long-standing BZDs

- Understand the patient's values and ensure they comprehend the risks of continued BZD use and the benefits of discontinuation.
- Offer reassurance about improved clarity and safety post-taper.
- Lower the dose by 10% to 25% every two to four weeks, with smaller reductions toward the end of the taper.
- Flexibility in the taper duration should be allowed but avoid reverting to previous higher doses (see *The Carlat Geriatric Psychiatry Report,* April/May/June 2022).

Anxiety-Reduction Techniques: Cognitive Restructuring and Relaxation in Older Adults

This fact sheet describes some key therapeutic techniques that are helpful in alleviating anxiety symptoms in older adults.

Cognitive Restructuring

Definition

Thoughts like, "I'll never be able to figure out how to use this computer," can give rise to negative feelings such as anxiety. A core component of cognitive behavioral therapy (CBT) focuses on identifying, challenging, and reframing these types of faulty beliefs.

Techniques

- *Identify automatic thoughts:* Listen for and point out negative thoughts occurring spontaneously and repeatedly. In CBT lingo, these are called "automatic thoughts."
  - People with anxiety may have thought patterns consisting of:
    - A belief that they cannot handle stressful or difficult situations.
    - A conviction that bad outcomes are likely to happen.
    - Fear of new opportunities or situations because of becoming overwhelmed or upset.
  - Examples of faulty thinking in older adults:
    - "I'm afraid of giving up my driver's license and having to rely on others for everything."
    - "All my friends are moving or passing on. I'll end up alone."
    - "The thought of moving out of my home and into assisted living terrifies me."
    - "I keep forgetting things; what if it's the start of Alzheimer's?"
- *Challenge dysfunctional beliefs:* work on developing healthier alternatives.
  - Example:
    - *Identify the anxious thought:*
      - "I can't make new friends at my age."
    - *Examine the evidence*
      - "What experiences have led you to think that making new friends is impossible?"
      - "How have you made friends in the past?"
    - *Challenge the thought*
      - "Is it possible that there are people who would value a new friendship as much as you would?"
      - "Could joining an activity, class, or community group lead to meeting people with similar interests?"
      - "Might there be ways to start with small steps, like saying hello or joining a conversation?"
    - *Develop a more balanced thought:* Work together to develop a more realistic thought after examining the belief. Have the patient say the new balanced thought out loud.
      - "While making new friends may feel challenging, I can take small steps to connect with others. There are people who would enjoy getting to know me, and I can focus on shared interests to build new friendships at my own pace."

Relaxation Skills

Definition

Techniques such as deep breathing exercises, progressive muscle relaxation, and positive imagery help manage the physiological symptoms of anxiety.

- Older adults can learn to use these techniques to reduce tension and promote relaxation.
- Encourage regular daily practice of these techniques, rather than using them only during moments of heightened anxiety when they may be less effective.

Techniques

Deep breathing exercises: Hyperventilation can trigger anxiety and panic. Teach patients to focus on slow, deep breaths to relax. Here's a helpful method from the United Kingdom's National Health Service:

- Stand, sit in a chair with back support, or lie down on a bed or yoga mat.
- Rearrange your clothing to make breathing easier.
- Breathe deeply into your belly.
- Inhale through your nose and exhale through your mouth.
- Keep your breathing gentle and steady.

- Count from one to five while inhaling and exhaling.
- Continue for at least five minutes.
- *Example:* An older adult with generalized anxiety disorder (GAD) may use deep breathing techniques to manage anticipatory anxiety before attending a medical appointment.

Progressive muscle relaxation (PMR)

PMR helps reduce anxiety-associated muscle tension by tensing and relaxing muscle groups. Here's a simplified guide:

- *Prepare*: Sit or lie in a comfortable position, close your eyes, and breathe deeply to begin relaxation.
- *Feet and legs:* Curl your toes downward, tense for 4 to 5 seconds, release, and feel the relaxation for 10 seconds. For calves, pretend to pull toes toward you, hold, then relax.
- *Hands and arms:* Clench hands into fists, tense for 4 to 5 seconds, release, and notice the relaxation for 10 seconds. Tense upper arms by bringing hands to shoulders, hold, then relax.
- *Shoulders and neck:* Lift shoulders to ears, hold the tension, and relax. Tilt head forward, hold, and release.
- *Face:* Squeeze eyes shut, wrinkle nose, clench teeth for four to five seconds, then relax into a natural expression.
- *Conclude:* Finish by taking deep breaths, enjoying the calmness and relaxation across your body.
- *Example:* PMR can be especially beneficial for older adults managing chronic pain and anxiety, as it helps to release tension in affected areas.

Positive imagery

Encourage patients to visualize calm and peaceful scenes, diverting attention from anxious thoughts. Patients should:

- Practice deep breathing during the exercise.
- Recall a happy memory or scene, such as a vacation spot, beach, mountain vista, or a pleasant memory of a person or situation.
- The person should fully describe the scene to themselves, making note of how it looks, sounds, smells, and feels, and the emotions it brings up.

Resources

Overall

- YouTube (www.youtube.com)
  - Description: YouTube has many high-quality, searchable videos for deep breathing, progressive muscle relaxation, and positive imagery.
  - Cost: Free

Deep breathing exercises

- Therapist Aid (https://tinyurl.com/47bneavt)
  - Description: A guided video for deep breathing along with worksheets is available.
  - Cost: Free

Progressive muscle relaxation (PMR)

- (https://tinyurl.com/3tyzstdx)
  - Description: A video walks patients through each stage of the technique.
  - Cost: Free

Guided imagery

- Dartmouth (https://tinyurl.com/4y9283tj)
  - Description: Offers guided audio recordings for several different scenarios.
  - Cost: Free

COMMON LATE-LIFE PSYCHIATRIC DISORDERS

Bipolar Disorder

Bipolar Disorder in Older Adults: Diagnosis

Bipolar disorder (BD) in older adults can present unique challenges and often differs from its presentation in younger individuals. This fact sheet aims to provide clinicians with information on identifying BD in older adults, focusing on its various presentations and unique features.

Epidemiology

- Older age bipolar disorder (OABD) impacts 0.5%–1% of community-dwelling older adults.
- However, it disproportionately accounts for 6% of geriatric psychiatry outpatient visits and 8%–10% of geriatric inpatient admissions, which speaks to the severity of the illness in later life.
- While onset of BD is associated with younger adults, 5%–10% of individuals with BD are 50 or older at the time of a first manic or hypomanic episode (Sajatovic M et al, *Bipolar Disord* 2015;17(7):689-704).

Diagnostic Criteria

- *Bipolar I disorder:* Characterized by at least one manic episode and often, but not necessarily, one or more major depressive episodes.
- *Bipolar II disorder:* Involves at least one hypomanic episode and one or more major depressive episodes.
- *Cyclothymic disorder:* Chronic fluctuations between hypomanic and depressive symptoms without meeting full criteria for either one, occurring for at least two years.

Four Types of Presentations in Older Adults

1. *Early-onset BD, now in older age*
   - This group comprises individuals diagnosed with BD at a younger age who have now aged into the older adult group.
   - Often, these individuals have experienced episodes of both mania and depression throughout their lives.
   - They are more likely to have a family history of BD and have higher rates of substance misuse.
   - Management involves utilizing a combination of mood stabilizers and second-generation antipsychotics, adjusted for age and medical comorbidities.
2. *Previously only had depression, now presenting with mania*
   - This cohort consists of patients with a history of depressive episodes and a prior diagnosis of unipolar depression, with no previous manic or hypomanic episodes.
   - Later in life, these patients present with their first manic episode. This is not as unusual as it sounds, as there can be a gap of up to 15 years between a first major depressive episode and a first manic episode (Shulman KI et al, *Am J Psychiatry* 1992;149(3):341–345).
   - In these cases, though, it is essential to evaluate for causes of secondary mania, which could be triggering the manic episode.
3. *New-onset mania triggered by a medical or neurological event (secondary mania)*
   - These individuals often have no prior history of affective illness.
   - Mania manifests following a significant medical event (eg, stroke, infection, medication side effect). Neurological illness is the most common cause of secondary mania (found in 36% of older adults with mania vs 8% of older adults without mania) (Shulman KI et al, 1992). See Table 6.
   - Older adults with secondary mania are more likely to have cognitive impairment. This can be mistaken for:
     - *Behavioral variant frontotemporal dementia (bvFTD)*
       - Both conditions may present with disinhibited behavior, hypersexuality, or significant personality changes.
       - Disinhibition in patients with bvFTD lacks the episodic nature typical of mania and is accompanied by pre-existing cognitive impairment.
       - Differentiating between the two can be challenging, especially if the patient presents with manic-like symptoms, confusion, and no prior psychiatric history.
       - Once symptoms subside, neuropsychological testing can aid in distinguishing bvFTD from OABD.
       - In OABD, cognitive and functional abilities typically return to baseline between episodes, whereas in people with bvFTD, impairments persist and progressively worsen.
     - *Delirium, hyperactive subtype:* Manic symptoms occurring alongside fluctuating levels of consciousness, active medical illness, and impaired attention are indicative of delirium rather than mania.
4. *Previously unrecognized or misdiagnosed BD*
   - These patients have had longstanding but unrecognized BD, which may have been misdiagnosed as anxiety, borderline personality disorder, ADHD, or irritability.

Table 6: **Causes of Secondary Mania in Older Adults**

Category	Specific Causes	Description
Infectious Diseases	Encephalitis	Inflammation of the brain, often due to infection, can cause psychiatric symptoms.
	HIV/AIDS	Neurological complications of HIV/AIDS may lead to mania.
	Neurosyphilis	Syphilis infection affecting the central nervous system can cause manic symptoms.
Medications	Antidepressants (especially TCAs, MAOIs)	Can elicit manic episodes in predisposed individuals.
	Antiparkinsonian medications (eg, levodopa, dopamine agonists—bromocriptine and pramipexole)	May induce mania via activation of dopamine.
	Immunosuppressants	High doses of corticosteroids, like prednisone, sometimes prompt mania.
	Some antibiotics and CV agents	Implicated meds include captopril, clarithromycin, and procainamide.
Metabolic and Nutritional Disorders	Cushing's syndrome	Excess cortisol production can cause psychiatric symptoms, like mania.
	Hyperthyroidism	An overactive thyroid might lead to increased metabolism and manic-like symptoms.
	Hyperparathyroidism	Elevated parathyroid hormone levels affect calcium metabolism and lead to mood disturbances.
	Hypothyroidism	An underactive thyroid can occasionally present with mixed or manic symptoms in older adults.
	Vitamin B12 deficiency	Deficiency leads to neurological and psychiatric symptoms, including mania.
Neurological Disorders	Brain tumors (diencephalic, frontal, hypothalamic)	Tumors can affect brain regions controlling mood and behavior.
	Multiple sclerosis	Demyelinating disease may cause neurological and psychiatric symptoms, including not uncommonly BD/mania.
	Temporal lobe epilepsy	Seizure disorders can impact mood regulation and lead to manic episodes.
	Traumatic brain injury (TBI)	Physical injury to the brain sometimes results in behavioral and mood changes.
	Stroke	Disruption of blood flow to the brain, especially on the right side of the frontal lobe, classically leads to manic symptoms.
Substance-Related Causes	Alcohol withdrawal	Sudden cessation of alcohol can result in withdrawal symptoms, comprising manic-like symptoms and/or hyperactive delirium.
	Drug misuse (eg, anabolic-androgenic steroids, amphetamines, cannabis, cocaine, high-dose caffeine, opioids, MDMA, PCP, synthetic cannabinoids)	Many stimulating illicit drugs can induce manic-like states.

Source: Larson EW and Richelson E, *Mayo Clin Proc* 1988;63(9):906-912.

Differences in History and Symptoms: Older Adults vs Younger Adults

Symptom onset

- Older adults are more likely to have OABD (onset after age 50).
- Younger adults typically experience onset in late adolescence or early adulthood.

Manic episodes

- Older adults may have more mixed episodes than euphoric mania.
- Manic symptoms in older adults often include irritability, aggression, and confusion.

Depressive episodes

- Depression is frequently more severe and prolonged in OABD.
- Somatic complaints (eg, pain, gastrointestinal issues) are more common in older adults.

Cognitive impairment

- Cognitive deficits are more prominent and can be mistaken for a neurocognitive disorder (eg, new-onset mania in late life can be mistaken for FTD [disinhibited behavior, hypersexuality, high-risk activities] or delirium, hyperactive subtype).
- Executive dysfunction, decreased cognitive flexibility, lower word fluency, and lower Mini-Mental State Examination scores are more commonly observed in OABD patients than in younger patients with BD (Schouws SN et al, *Am J Geriatr Psychiatry* 2009;17(6):508-15).
- Brain imaging findings include:
  - Increased white matter hyperintensities and cerebrovascular impairment in patients with OABD.
  - Increased right-hemispheric lesions, predominantly in the frontal lobe, temporal lobe, fusiform gyrus, and thalamus in patients with mania due to a brain injury (Barahona-Corrêa JB et al, *Transl Psychiatry* 2020).

PRACTICE POINT: *Encourage all patients with OABD to strictly control vascular risk factors and follow up routinely with their physicians.*

Table 7: **Differences in Bipolar Disorder Presentations**

Feature	Younger Adults	Older Adults
Onset	Teens to early 20s	After age 50
Family History	Common	Less common
Course	Episodic, higher recurrence	Persistent, slower resolution
Substance Abuse	Higher prevalence	Lower prevalence
Cognitive Impairment	Less common	More common
Neurological Findings	Less consistent	More consistent abnormalities
Psychotic Features	More prevalent	Less prevalent
Depressive Episodes	Less prevalent	More prevalent
Mortality Rate	Lower	Higher
Suicide Risk	Higher	Lower
Medical Comorbidity	Less common	More common

Source: Sajatovic M et al, *Bipolar Disord* 2015.

Bipolar Disorder in Older Adults: Treatment Overview

This fact sheet provides an overview for the treatment of different stages in bipolar disorder (BD) in older adults. Unfortunately, few large-scale studies have been done in this population, so in many cases recommendations have been extrapolated from younger adults.

Psychopharmacological Strategies

- The initial trial of medication for mania, hypomania, or depression should last at least 3–4 weeks.
- Consider a judicious combination of medications if monotherapy does not yield the desired results. Most older adults (82%) will be stabilized on two or more psychotropic medications (Rej S et al, *Int J Geriatr Psychiatry* 2017;32(12):1459–1465).
- Once an older adult responds to treatment, continue it for 6–12 months to prevent recurrence of a mood episode.
- For patients in remission, a gradual reduction and discontinuation of medications can be attempted after 12 months, though in many cases patients will require chronic maintenance therapy.

Psychosocial Interventions

- *Cognitive behavioral therapy (CBT):* Effective in reducing residual symptoms of depression.
- *Interpersonal and social rhythm therapy (IPSRT):* Focuses on establishing daily routines and improving interpersonal functioning. IPSRT has not been studied in older adults but would likely be beneficial.
- *Medication adherence skills training*: Assists with medication management and medication adherence. This is an important issue to discuss with patients and families, as 55% of older adults with BD become nonadherent, often resulting in recurrence of depression (Depp CA et al, *Bipolar Disord* 2007;9(6):636-s45).
- *Physical activity:* Improves mood and overall health.
- *Psychoeducation:* Inform patients and caregivers about the disorder, treatment options, and early warning signs of an impending mood episode.
- *Sleep hygiene:* Encourage regular sleep patterns and avoidance of caffeine and electronics before bed. Disrupted sleep or irregular sleep schedules can trigger mood episodes.
- *Support groups:* Provide a platform for patients and caregivers to share experiences and strategies.

Initial Assessment

- *Comprehensive history and physical examination*
  - Include psychiatric, medical, and family history.
  - Evaluate for secondary causes of mania (eg, medications, metabolic disturbances).
- *Medication review*
  - Screen for drug-drug interactions and medications contributing to mood symptoms (eg, corticosteroids, stimulants).
- *Laboratory tests*
  - Complete blood count (CBC), comprehensive metabolic panel (CMP), thyroid stimulating hormone (TSH), and vitamin B12 & folate.
  - Additional tests to consider include fasting lipid panel to monitor for metabolic risks associated with antipsychotics, hemoglobin A1c, vitamin D, RPR, HIV, urine toxicology screen, ECG for medication monitoring, and neuroimaging.
- *Cognitive assessment*
  - Baseline assessment to differentiate BD symptoms from dementia or delirium.

Acute Treatment of Mania

First-line medications

- *Lithium*
  - Target serum level: 0.5–0.8 mEq/L in older adults.
  - Monitor closely for toxicity due to reduced renal clearance in older adults.
- *Valproate*
  - Preferred for patients who are intolerant to lithium or experiencing a mixed episode.
- *Second-generation antipsychotics (SGAs)*
  - Effective options: Quetiapine, risperidone, olanzapine.

Additional therapies

- *Carbamazepine*
  - Consider for atypical BD or secondary mania (Sajatovic M and Chen P, *Psychiatr Clin N Am* 2011;34(2):319–333).

- *Electroconvulsive Therapy (ECT)*
  - Indicated for severe mania, refractory symptoms, or patients with high suicide risk.
- *Benzodiazepines*
  - Short-term use (eg, clonazepam, lorazepam) at doses 25%–50% lower than for younger adults can help with acute manic symptoms.
- *Psychotherapy*
  - Consider supportive therapy or CBT for adjunctive management.

Acute Treatment of Bipolar Depression

First-line medications

- *Lamotrigine*
  - Gradual dose titration to minimize rash risk.
- *Quetiapine*
  - Effective for depressive episodes at low to moderate doses.
- *Lurasidone*
  - Can be used as monotherapy or as an adjunct to mood stabilizers.
- *Olanzapine/fluoxetine combination*
  - Particularly useful in severe or refractory depression.

Combination therapy

- *Mood stabilizers with antidepressants*
  - The addition of bupropion or SSRIs (eg, sertraline, escitalopram) should be approached cautiously in patients with bipolar disorder due to the risk of inducing mania or a mixed episode. Antidepressants are best used in combination with a mood stabilizer to reduce this risk, particularly in bipolar I disorder.
  - Avoid prescribing antidepressants for patients who have rapid cycling or mixed features.

Additional therapies

- ECT
  - Effective for severe/refractory depression or depression with psychotic features.
- Psychotherapy
  - Consider CBT or IPSRT.

Treatment of Hypomania

Medications

- *Mood stabilizers*
  - Lithium or valproate.
- *SGAs*
  - Quetiapine, risperidone.

Additional interventions

- *Lifestyle modifications*
  - Structured routines and sleep hygiene.
- *Benzodiazepines*
  - Short-term use for agitation or insomnia, with doses 25–50% lower than in adults.

Treatment of Mixed Episodes

Medications

- *Valproate*
  - Preferred due to efficacy in mixed states.
- *SGAs*
  - Effective options: Aripiprazole, olanzapine.

Additional therapies

- *ECT*
  - Indicated for severe or refractory mixed episodes.
- *Psychotherapy*
  - CBT

Maintenance Treatment

Medications

- *Lithium*
  - Established long-term effectiveness for both mania and depression relapse prevention.
- *Lamotrigine*
  - Ideal for depression relapse prevention, especially in patients intolerant to lithium.
- *SGAs*
  - Quetiapine, aripiprazole, olanzapine.

Additional therapies

- *CBT*
  - Targets residual symptoms and promotes coping strategies.
- *Regular physical activity*
  - Reduces mood symptoms and improves overall well-being.
- *Psychoeducation*
  - For both patients and caregivers and to promote medication adherence.
- *Sleep regulation*
  - Prevents mood destabilization.
- *ECT for maintenance*
  - Consider in recurrent severe episodes.

Bipolar Disorder in Older Adults: Mood Stabilizers

The use of mood stabilizers in older adults requires careful consideration due to age-related pharmacokinetic changes, medical comorbidities, and polypharmacy risks.

Lithium

Benefits

- *Anti-suicide properties:* Reduces suicide risk across all ages in both unipolar and bipolar depression. Given the high rate of death by suicide in older adults, this is an important advantage (D'Souza R et al, *Curr Psychiatry Rep* 2011;13:488–492).
- *Efficacy:* More effective in treating mania than divalproex (Young RC et al, *Am J Psychiatry* 2017;174(11):1086–1093).
- *Cognitive protection:* Potentially reduces dementia risk due to neuroprotective properties. Even at subtherapeutic concentrations (0.25–0.5 mEq/L), older adults taking lithium have had better performance on memory and attention tests (Forlenza FV et al, *Br J Psychiatry* 2019;215(5):668–674).

Risks

- *Side effects:* Delirium (higher risk in older adults compared to younger adults), cognitive impairment, ataxia, weight gain, edema, tremor, acne, worsening of psoriasis.
- *Serious concerns:* Hypothyroidism, nephrotoxicity, nephrogenic diabetes insipidus (characterized by increased urine frequency and thirst), sick sinus syndrome (avoid using in older adults with cardiovascular disease).
- *Toxicity*
  - Higher risk due to decreased renal function in older adults and potential drug interactions (eg, thiazide diuretics, nonsteroidal anti-inflammatory drugs, angiotensin-converting enzyme inhibitors).
  - Signs: Coarse tremor, nausea, vomiting, diarrhea, ataxia, confusion, renal failure, seizures, coma.
  - Treatment
    - Discontinue lithium immediately.
    - Ensure hydration to enhance renal clearance of lithium.
    - Monitor lithium levels, renal function, and electrolytes.
    - Patients with moderate to severe toxicity may require admission to a medical unit for supportive care, IV fluids, treatment of electrolyte disturbances, managing seizures, and cardiac monitoring.
    - Hemodialysis is indicated in severe cases when lithium levels are over 4.0 mEq/L or if renal function is significantly compromised.

Dosing

- Recommend doses 25%–50% lower than those used in adults. Aim for target serum levels of 0.5-0.8 mEq/L.
- Initial dose: 300 mg qHS, ranging from 300–900 mg qHS.
- Sustained release preparations and once nightly dosing are recommended. This can decrease peak levels, protecting the kidneys and improving tolerability.

Divalproex/Valproic Acid

Benefits

- *Tolerance:* Generally, well tolerated in older adults without dementia. In patients with dementia, medium to high doses have been linked with neurotoxicity (Tariot PN et al, *Arch Gen Psychiatry* 2011;68(8):853-861).
- *Efficacy:* Particularly useful for rapid-cycling bipolar disorder.

Risks

- *Common side effects:* Nausea, sedation, weight gain.
- *Serious concerns:* Hepatotoxicity, hyperammonemia (confusion), thrombocytopenia, pancreatitis, parkinsonism. Hepatotoxicity and pancreatitis are less common in older adults. Thrombocytopenia occurs more frequently in older adults.

Dosing

- Lower doses are recommended due to decreased protein binding and longer half-life in older adults.
- *Initial dose:* 250 mg qHS, with a range of 500–1000 mg daily
- *Therapeutic range:* 65–90 mg/L (Chen ST et al, *J Clin Psychiatry* 1999;60(3):181-186).

Carbamazepine

Benefits

- Often a last resort choice in older adults because of its side effects and limited evidence of benefit.

- It may help individuals with nonclassical features of bipolar disorder (BD). These include continuous cycling, high irritability, comorbid substance misuse and anxiety, mood-incongruent delusions, and a negative first-degree family history of mood disorders (Post RM, *Psychiatr Clin North Am* 2016;39(1):11–33).

Risks

- *Side effects:* Ataxia, dizziness, fatigue, headache, sedation, nausea, vomiting, blurred vision.
- *Serious concerns:* Agranulocytosis, aplastic anemia, atrioventricular conduction delays (QTc prolongation), hyponatremia (syndrome of inappropriate antidiuretic hormone, or SIADH), rashes, urinary retention. Changes in blood counts (agranulocytosis, aplastic anemia) can occur more frequently in older adults.
- *Drug interactions:* Significant CYP3A induction leads to reduced blood levels of up to 25% of medications, including carbamazepine (also metabolized by CYP3A4). Induction can have a significant effect on lowering the levels of blood thinners like apixaban and warfarin.

Dosing

- *Initial dose:* 100 mg daily or BID, gradually increasing to 400–800 mg daily. Because of autoinduction, the dosage may need to be increased again after 4–6 weeks.
- *Therapeutic range:* 4–12 μg/L

Lamotrigine

Benefits

- *Depression prevention:* More effective than lithium in preventing bipolar depression. Poor at treating or preventing mania. For people with BD-I, it is often added to another mood stabilizer or second-generation antipsychotic for control of mania.
- *Tolerance:* Fewer cognitive side effects compared to other anticonvulsants.

Risks

- *Side effects:* Nausea, insomnia, sedation, back pain, rash.
- *Serious concerns:* Rare cases of Stevens-Johnson syndrome (SJS), especially when combined with valproate. SJS symptoms include widespread and confluent rash, involvement of mucosal membranes, and systemic signs such as high fever and elevated white blood cell count. If any of the above develop, discontinue lamotrigine and recommend patient be evaluated in the emergency department.

Dosing

Initial dose: 25 mg daily, with a range of 100–200 mg daily. Increased by 25 mg every other week.

Gabapentin

Considerations

- *Not a true mood stabilizer:* Lacks efficacy in treating mania or depression.
- *Uses:* Helpful for alcohol use disorder, anxiety, neuropathic pain, and restless legs syndrome in older adults.

Oxcarbazepine

Considerations

- *SIADH risk:* High rate of hyponatremia, up to 50% in some studies, limits its usefulness in older adults.
- *Efficacy:* Limited evidence in treating late-life bipolar disorder.

Table 8: **Commonly Prescribed Mood Stabilizers in Older Adults**

Medication	Initial Dose	Dose Range	Reference Range	Evidence	FDA-Approved Indications	Common Side Effects	Serious Side Effects	Dose Titration	Considerations in Older Adults
Carbamazepine	100 mg daily or BID	400–800 mg/d	4–12 µg/L	Very low	Acute manic/ mixed (Equetro), bipolar 1 disorder, seizures, trigeminal neuralgia	Ataxia, blurred vision, dizziness, fatigue, headache, nausea, sedation, vomiting	Agranulocytosis, aplastic anemia, atrioventricular conduction delays, hyponatremia, rashes, urinary retention	Increase by 100–200 mg every 1–2 weeks	• Significant drug-drug interactions due to CYP3A induction • Higher risk of neurotoxic effects and blood count changes in older adults • Regularly monitor blood counts, sodium, liver enzymes, and electrolytes
Divalproex	250 mg PO qHS	500– 1000 mg/d	65–90 mg/L	Low	Acute mania; bipolar disorder; partial, complex, and absence seizures	Nausea, sedation, weight gain	Hepatotoxicity, hyperammonemia, pancreatitis, parkinsonism thrombocytopenia	Increase by 250 mg every 1–2 weeks	• In patients with dementia, it might be more helpful for disinhibition than agitation or aggression • Lower doses recommended in older adults due to decreased protein binding and longer half-life • Medium to high doses in patients with dementia may be neurotoxic • Greater risk of thrombocytopenia in older adults • Regularly monitor liver function and platelets • Check ammonia levels if patient develops altered mental status
Lamotrigine	25 mg daily	100–200 mg/d	N/A	Low	Bipolar 1 disorder, maintenance, seizures	Back pain, insomnia, nausea, sedation, rash	Stevens-Johnson syndrome (SJS)	Increase by 25 mg every 2 weeks	• Generally, well tolerated with less chance of cognitive side effects • Caution with concomitant use of valproate due to higher risk of SJS • Regular monitoring for skin reactions, especially during initial treatment
Lithium	300 mg qHS	300– 900 mg qHS	0.5–0.8 mEq/L	Low	Acute mania/ mixed and maintenance; bipolar 1 disorder	Acne, ataxia, cognitive impairment, edema, psoriasis exacerbation, tremor, weight gain	Hypothyroidism, nephrotoxicity, nephrogenic diabetes insipidus, sick sinus syndrome, toxicity	Increase by 300 mg every 1–2 weeks	• Anti-suicide effect • May prevent dementia • Higher risk of side effects and toxicity due to declining renal function and greater risk of drug interactions in older adults • Regularly monitor thyroid, renal function, and calcium

Table 9: **Monitoring Recommendations for Divalproex, Lithium, and Carbamazepine**

Parameter	Depakote (Divalproex)	Lithium	Carbamazepine
Baseline Tests			
CBC	Yes	Yes	Yes
Liver Function Tests (LFTs)	Yes	No	Yes
Renal Function Tests	No	Yes	Yes
Thyroid Function Tests	No	Yes	No
Electrolytes	Yes	Yes	Yes
ECG	No	Yes (if cardiovascular risk)	Yes (monitor QTc interval)
Ongoing Monitoring			
Weight/BMI	Every 6 months	Every 6–12 months	Every 6–12 months
CBC	Every 6 months	Every 6–12 months	Every 6 months
Electrolytes	Every 6–12 months	Every 3–6 months	Every 6–12 months
Renal Function Tests	No	Every 3–6 months	Every 6–12 months
Liver Function Tests (LFTs)	Every 6–12 months	No	Every 6–12 months
Ammonia Levels	If confusion occurs	No	No
Thyroid Function Tests	No	Every 6–12 months	No
Serum Drug Levels	2 weeks after initiation/dose change, then every 6–12 months	5–7 days after initiation/dose change, then every 3-6 months	3–5 days after initiation/dose change, dose may need adjustment as CBZ induces its own metabolism, then every 6-12 months
ECG	No	Annually (if cardiovascular risk)	Every 6–12 months (if cardiac risk)

COMMON LATE-LIFE PSYCHIATRIC DISORDERS

Depressive Disorders

Depression in Older Adults: Diagnosis

Late-life depression (LLD) is defined as a depressive episode occurring in an individual aged 60 or older. It impacts about 2%–5% of older adults in the community (Steffens DC et al, *Arch Gen Psychiatry* 2000;57(6):601-607). In medical and skilled nursing settings, LLD occurs in up to 25% of older adults. While the clinical interview remains the gold standard for diagnosis, LLD is frequently overlooked or misattributed to normal aging or anxiety. It is important to note that even subthreshold depressive symptoms can lead to significant disability and may warrant treatment.

Clinical Presentation

In younger adults, depression is diagnosed by the presence of low mood or loss of interest or pleasure plus four out of eight of the classic SIGECAPS symptoms occurring over a two-week span. While these criteria are also applicable in older adults, there are some variations and special considerations.

- ***M****ood*
  - "How have your spirits been over the last two weeks?"
  - "Have you felt so down that your entire life has been affected?"
  - Some older adults will not endorse feeling "depressed," but will admit to:
    - Having low spirits
    - Feeling sad
    - Increased irritability
    - Being discouraged
    - Never feeling happy
    - Becoming desperate
  - Other patients will feel a constant sense of "nervousness" or "anxiety" but on further assessment, they will have LLD rather than an anxiety disorder.
- ***S****leep*
  - "How have you slept over the last two weeks?"
  - The most common complaints are difficulty falling asleep and frequent nighttime awakenings. Patients may have early-morning awakenings but as a result of age-related changes in sleeping patterns, instead of depression.
- ***I****nterest decrease*
  - "Have you found any activities enjoyable lately?"
  - Look for signs like social withdrawal, neglecting hobbies/friends, or a lack of enthusiasm for activities formerly enjoyed.
- ***G****uilt*
  - "Do you feel that you are a good person?"
  - "Have you felt guilty about things you've done or haven't done?"
- ***E****nergy decrease*
  - "How has your energy level been over the last couple of weeks?"
  - "Is it taking longer than usual for you to get things done?"
  - Rather than decreased energy, older adults with depression frequently report weariness.
- **C**oncentration
  - "Do you forget names, addresses, or birthdays?"
  - Older adults with LLD are more likely to present with memory problems than with the concentration issues seen in younger adults. Specific memory complaints include increased forgetfulness, trouble finding the right words, difficulty reasoning through decisions, and slowed thinking.
- ***A****ppetite decrease*
  - "Have you felt like eating?
  - "Have you lost weight lately?"
  - Older adults rarely gain weight because of depression. Significant weight loss is a major concern since it can lead to frailty, from which some older adults never recover. Recommend adding Ensure® or BOOST® to the meals of patients who have lost considerable weight.
- ***P****sychomotor retardation or agitation*
  - This is usually assessed more by observation than by asking questions, but you can ask, "Have you noticed any slowing down in your movements or speech?" or "Have you felt unusually restless or agitated?"
  - Patients who have psychomotor retardation will describe slowness. With psychomotor agitation, complaints center around nervousness, agita, and insomnia.
- ***S****uicidality*

  - "Have you had thoughts of wishing you were dead?"
  - "Have you been thinking about ways to end your life?"
  - Older adults endorse suicidal thoughts less often compared to their younger counterparts but have more thoughts of death and dying. Hopelessness and worthlessness are major red flags that an older adult may be thinking of suicide. See "Suicide Risk in Older Adults: Assessment and Management" [page 46] fact sheet in the Depressive Disorders section of this book.

Other Aspects of Depression Common in Older Adults

Cognitive impairment

- Cognitive impairment due to depression begins acutely and with the onset of the depressive episode. In contrast, dementia has a slowly progressive, insidious course that at times might include periods of depression.
- Conduct a cognitive screen on any older adult with depression and follow them closely for the possible emergence of dementia once their depression improves, since depression is a risk factor for dementia.

Grief

Ask about grieving and try to distinguish acute grief symptoms from depression (though the presence of grief does not automatically exclude major depression).

Medication Effects

Commonly used agents that can cause depression or other mood changes are angiotensin-converting enzyme inhibitors, beta-blockers, calcium-channel blockers, corticosteroids, levetiracetam, metoclopramide, and opioids.

Psychotic depression

- Psychosis is much more likely to accompany depression in older adults than in younger patients. It can occur in up to 45% of older adults hospitalized with depression. Assess for persecutory, nihilistic, or hypochondriacal—often focused on gastrointestinal function—delusions (Kessing LV, *Int J Geriatr Psychiatry* 2006;21(12):1127-1131).
- While less common than delusions, hallucinations can have a significant impact in older adults.

Somatic symptoms

- Older adults with depression often complain of increased pain or stomach issues.
- Other somatic symptoms, like changes in energy or sleep, overlap with the effects of medications and comorbid disease.
- LLD can also be triggered by medical conditions such as heart disease, diabetes, Parkinson's disease, strokes, and cancer.

Assessment

- *Steps in assessment*
  - The clinical interview is the gold standard of assessment (see "Clinical Presentation" section above).
  - Obtain collateral history from a family member or caregiver.
  - Assess nutritional status, functional status, medical history, and current medications.
  - Screen for cognitive dysfunction (Montreal Cognitive Assessment, Mini-Mental Status Exam, Saint Louis University Mental Status Exam).
- *Tools*
  - The Geriatric Depression Scale (GDS):
    - The short form has 15 yes/no questions that focus on psychological rather than physical symptoms and takes three to four minutes to complete.
    - The GDS has a sensitivity of 85% with specificity of 75% (Mitchell AJ et al, *Am J Geriatr Psychiatry* 2010;18(12):1066–1077).
    - The GDS is available in the public domain: https://tinyurl.com/mry4dwha.
  - The Patient Health Questionnaire-9 (PHQ-9) is another commonly used instrument to assess depression but is not specific to older adults.
  - Laboratory tests to rule out other causes of LLD:
    - Complete blood count (CBC), Chem 10, LFTs.
    - Free T4 and TSH, U/A, Utox, Vitamin B12, and folate levels.
    - Rapid plasma reagin and HIV if appropriate.
    - Head CT or brain MRI, especially for cases of late-onset depression.
    - EEG/PET/SPECT if indicated.

Suicide Risk in Older Adults: Assessment and Management

Older adults account for 19% of deaths from suicide in the US, despite being only 15% of the population. As a result, suicidal thoughts in older adults require immediate attention. Be especially careful with elderly white men who have suicidal thoughts, as their rate of death by suicide is four times higher than the rest of the population.

Assessment

- Older adults are less likely to spontaneously report thoughts of suicide and should be asked specifically about them.
- While some older adults may be put off by these questions, asking about suicide will not trigger an attempt and may help to save someone's life.
- I try to normalize questions by starting off with, "Unfortunately, rates of suicide have been climbing since the pandemic. Because of this, I talk to everyone about it."
- Some questions to ask are:
  - "Have you ever wished you were dead or that you could go to sleep and never wake up again?"
  - "Have you had thoughts about ending your life?"

  If "YES":
  - "Have you thought about how you might do it?"
  - "How likely are you to try to do something?"
  - "Have you worked out a plan?"

  If "YES":
  - "Have you done anything, researched methods, or prepared anything to help you?"
- Common means of suicide in older adults include firearms, hanging, self-poisoning, and falls from a height. Ask about:
  - Availability of firearms.
  - Attempts at hanging (eg, tying a noose or buying ropes).
  - Collecting/hoarding pills.
  - Scouting locations by visiting nearby tall buildings, parking garages, or bridges.

Risk Factors for Suicide

- Evaluating risk factors can guide your next steps, including determining whether hospitalization is necessary for someone at high or moderate risk.
- Standard suicide screens for adults focus on physical symptoms such as trouble sleeping, but many older adults will have these symptoms anyway because of comorbid medical conditions, medication side effects, or age-related changes.
- Instead, I recommend also focusing on psychological factors. IS PATH WARM is a useful mnemonic for warning signs of suicide (Lester D et al, *Psychol Rep* 2011;108(2):402–404).
  - **I**deation: Talking about death; planning for ways to hurt oneself.
  - **S**ubstance abuse: Increased alcohol or drug use.
  - **P**urposelessness: No reason for living; no sense of purpose.
  - **A**nxiety: Agitated, anxious, unable to sleep.
  - **T**rapped: Feeling trapped, like there is no way out.
  - **H**opelessness: Loss of hope that the situation will improve.
  - **W**ithdrawal: Withdrawal from friends, family, or society; neglecting self-care.
  - **A**nger: Anger, rage, revenge-seeking.
  - **R**ecklessness: Acting reckless, engaging in risky behavior.
  - **M**ood changes: Psychiatric illness is present in most older adults who die by suicide.
- Immediate intervention is crucial for high-risk older adults with suicidal ideation, particularly those with untreated conditions, such as depression and chronic pain, as well as those who have a history of suicide attempts; access to lethal means; significant life stressors; few or no confidants; or a reluctance to seek mental health care. The presence of hopelessness or a specific suicide plan also greatly increases the urgency for action.

CASE VIGNETTE: *Mr. Harrison, an 82-year-old widower, presents to the clinic after his daughter found a note expressing hopelessness and "not wanting to be a burden." He reports passive suicidal ideation, insomnia, significant weight loss, and withdrawal from social activities over the past six months. His medical history includes recent functional decline due to osteoarthritis and macular degeneration, contributing to his social isolation. Risk assessment identifies key factors: advanced age, male gender, chronic illness, social isolation, and loss of a spouse, while protective factors include a supportive daughter and religious beliefs. He denies active intent but has researched overdose methods. Immediate management involves voluntary hospitalization for stabilization and safety, initiating sertraline 25 mg/day, and addressing grief and functional decline through psychotherapy and occupational therapy.*

Risk Management

Immediate

- *Collaborative safety planning:* If there is an immediate risk, ensure the safety of the individual, which might involve voluntary or involuntary hospitalization.
  - Do not leave the person alone until they are in a safe environment.
  - If the person is sent home, rely on licensed professionals instead of family/caregivers to keep the patient safe.
  - Secure firearms or access to other lethal means. In some jurisdictions, police may have the authority to confiscate weapons. Otherwise, ask that firearms be kept in a gun safe/locker to which the patient doesn't have access, or taken for safe keeping by family or friends.
- *Family and caregiver involvement:* Engage family members and caregivers in the assessment and decision-making process.
- *Multidisciplinary collaboration:* Collaborate with other healthcare professionals to ensure everyone is in the loop and that comprehensive care addressing the patient's physical, psychological, and social needs is provided.

Ongoing

- *Address modifiable risk factors*
  - Identify and address underlying stressors such as chronic pain, untreated medical illness, poor sleep quality, visual impairment, functional impairment, bereavement, or social isolation that may be contributing to suicidal thoughts.
  - Promote meaningful activities, social interactions, and hobbies that foster a sense of purpose, connectedness, and enjoyment. These can serve as protective factors against suicidal thoughts.
- *Psychotherapy:* Offer evidence-based psychotherapeutic interventions such as cognitive behavioral therapy, dialectical behavior therapy, or interpersonal therapy. These modalities can address underlying psychological distress, maladaptive thought patterns, and interpersonal conflicts contributing to thoughts of self-harm.
- *Medication management*
  - Consider pharmacotherapy, particularly selective serotonin reuptake inhibitors (SSRIs) or serotonin-norepinephrine reuptake inhibitors (SNRIs). Antidepressants have demonstrated efficacy in reducing suicidal ideation and improving mood in older adults with depression.
  - Other life-saving interventions to consider are lithium in patients with either bipolar disorder or major depressive disorder; clozapine in patients with schizophrenia; and electroconvulsive therapy or esketamine for rapid relief of suicidal thoughts.
- *Regular follow-up*
  - Implement a structured follow-up schedule to monitor the patient's response to treatment, assess suicide risk, and adjust interventions as needed.
  - Close monitoring is crucial during the initial phases of treatment and dosage adjustments.
- *Education and support for caregivers:* Provide education and support for family members and caregivers to help them understand the patient's condition, recognize warning signs of suicidal thinking, and implement strategies to promote safety and supportive environments.
- *Emergency response protocol:* Establish clear protocols for managing acute suicidal crises, including procedures for hospitalization, crisis intervention, and coordination with emergency services when necessary, including utilizing **988**, the national suicide and crisis lifeline.

Antidepressants in Older Adults

Medication Classes (in order of preference)

Selective serotonin reuptake inhibitors (SSRIs)

- SSRIs are the first-line treatment for late-life depression (LLD) because of their favorable side effect profiles and because they also help with frequent co-occurring anxiety.
- Start with
  - Sertraline at 25 mg daily and titrate up to 50–200 mg per response.
  - Escitalopram at 5 mg daily and titrate up to 20 mg. Although citalopram has more efficacy data, I avoid it due to its boxed warning for QTc prolongation at doses > 20 mg/day in older adults.
- All serotonergic antidepressants can cause
  - Bleeding, especially in those also taking nonsteroidal anti-inflammatory drugs, anticoagulants, or antiplatelet agents. For patients prescribed blood thinners, I recommend clearing the SSRI/serotonin norepinephrine reuptake inhibitor (SNRI) with the patient's primary care physician.
  - Decreased bone density, which causes a higher risk of fractures. If a patient has a history of falls or fractures, I will choose mirtazapine or bupropion first-line.
  - Rates of hyponatremia with SSRIs/SNRIs are relatively high in older adults. Hyponatremia occurs within 14 days of medication initiation. Monitor sodium levels closely when starting or changing dosages. Bupropion and mirtazapine have lower rates of hyponatremia than SSRIs (Nelson JC, *Handb Exp Pharmacol* 2019;250:389–413).
- Drug-drug interactions
  - For patients taking other medications, consider escitalopram, mirtazapine, sertraline, or venlafaxine, as they are the least likely to interact.

SNRIs

SNRIs cause more side effects, including falls, than SSRIs in older adults, and so are second-line treatments, though may be a preferred option in people with comorbid pain (Sobieraj DM et al, *J Am Geriatr Soc* 2019;67(8):1571-1581).

Other antidepressants

- *Bupropion* is a stimulating antidepressant that can also assist with anhedonia, apathy, and smoking cessation.
- *Mirtazapine* was my go-to choice, but recent findings suggest it may carry a higher risk of adverse outcomes compared to sertraline. As a result, it is now my third-line option (Ishtiak-Ahmed K et al, *Am J Psychiatry* 2024;181(1):47–56). Its side effects, such as sedation and appetite stimulation, can be beneficial for addressing insomnia and weight loss, common concerns among older adults.
- *Tricyclic antidepressants* have efficacy in LLD but, along with monoamine oxidase inhibitors, are not recommended due to their potential for drug-drug interactions and poor side effect profiles.
- *Vilazodone* has excellent safety and tolerability. It also treats anxiety.
- *Vortioxetine* holds promise in LLD due to its pro-cognitive benefits, which may extend beyond its antidepressant effects.
- *Other treatments* include electroconvulsive therapy (ECT), transcranial magnetic stimulation (TMS), ketamine, and esketamine.

Augmentation

- Augment (in order of preference) with aripiprazole, mirtazapine, bupropion XL, quetiapine (Lenze EJ and Oughli AH, *J Am Geriatr Soc* 2019;67(8):1555–1556), or methylphenidate.
- Aripiprazole augmentation of 2–15 mg/day can result in remission in 44% vs 29% of people taking placebo (Lenze EJ et al, *Lancet* 2015;386(10011):2404–2412). In older adults with treatment-resistant depression, augmentation of an antidepressant with aripiprazole is significantly better than switching to bupropion (Lenze EJ et al, *N Engl J Med* 2023;388(12):1067-1079). But be aware that aripiprazole causes more akathisia than placebo (26% vs 12%) and more parkinsonism than placebo (17% vs 2%) (Lenze EJ et al, *Lancet* 2015;386).
- Methylphenidate augmentation of 5–40 mg/day can improve mood, boost well-being, and lead to higher remission rates. It appears to be a safe strategy, though you should first consult with a cardiologist for patients with cardiac risk factors. We do not have much data on methylphenidate's long-term use, though it might be safe for up to six months. Consider prescribing it short-term to help "jump-start" recovery (Lavretsky H et al, *Am J Psychiatry* 2015;172(6):561–569; Mintzer et al, *JAMA Neurol* 2021;78(11):1324-1332).

Major Depressive Disorder with Psychotic Features

This is one of the few situations in geriatric psychiatry in which polypharmacy is recommended from the beginning. To the primary antidepressant, consider adding aripiprazole, quetiapine, or olanzapine.

If Antidepressant Treatment Fails, Consider the Following

- *Adherence:* A common reason for low antidepressant effectiveness is that many patients never take them, stop them early, or take them intermittently.

- *Suboptimal trial duration*: Older adults may respond to antidepressants more slowly than younger adults, possibly requiring 10–12 weeks before effects are seen.
- *Suboptimal dose:* While the adage is to "start low," remember to keep going and use the full dosage range of the drug (Lenze EJ and Oughli AH, *J Am Geriatr Soc* 2019).
- *Too long on an ineffective treatment:* If the first treatment is unsuccessful, switch to the next option (Srifuengfung M et al, *Ther Adv Psychopharmacol* 2023;13:1–14).
- *Broadening treatment strategy:* Antidepressants tend to be less effective in older adults than in younger adults, with response rates of approximately 50% in older adults compared to 60%–70% in younger adults (Gutsmiedl K et al, *BMC Psychiatry* 2020;20(1):102). When initial antidepressant treatment is unsuccessful, a comprehensive approach is recommended. This may involve combining medication with nonpharmacological interventions such as regular exercise, social activities, dietary modifications, and psychotherapy.

Treatment Algorithm

- *Mild depression:* Psychotherapy OR pharmacotherapy
- *Moderate depression:* Psychotherapy AND pharmacotherapy.
- *Severe depression without psychotic features:* Psychotherapy and pharmacotherapy, OR ECT.
- *Severe depression with psychotic features:* Pharmacotherapy with antidepressant and antipsychotic, OR ECT.
- *Treatment-resistant depression:* Augmentation, OR switching drug classes, OR ECT/TMS/VNS, OR other treatments.

Table 10: **Antidepressant Medications and Dosing Guidelines for Older Adults**

Drug Class/Drug	Starting Dose	Dose Range	Comments
SSRIs			
Escitalopram	5 mg daily	10–20 mg daily	• Bleeding risk • Hyponatremia • Few drug-drug interactions
Sertraline	12.5–25 mg daily	50–200 mg daily	• Bleeding risk • Drug-drug interactions at doses > 150 mg/day • Hyponatremia
SNRIs			
Duloxetine	20 mg daily	60–90 mg daily	• Activating • Bleeding risk • Discontinuation syndrome • Dose-dependent increases in blood pressure and heart rate • Hyponatremia • Urinary retention • Useful for co-occurring pain
Venlafaxine ER	37.5 mg qAM	75–225 mg daily	• Same as for duloxetine • Few drug-drug interactions
Other antidepressants			
Bupropion	75 mg qAM	150 mg BID in the morning and early afternoon with the SR formulation or 150–300 mg qAM with the XL formulation	• Activating • Do not order if history of seizures, eating disorders, or alcohol use disorder • May worsen anxiety or insomnia • Might improve apathy • Smoking cessation
Mirtazapine	7.5 mg qHS	15–30 mg qHS	• Caution in renal/hepatic impairment • Sedation • Weight gain
Vortioxetine	5 mg daily	5–20 mg daily	• Bleeding risk • Fewer sexual side effects • Hyponatremia • Nausea • Potential cognitive-enhancing effects
Vilazodone	10 mg daily	20–40 mg daily	• Bleeding risk • Hyponatremia • Less weight gain and sexual side effects • Nausea • Take with food
Augmentation			
Aripiprazole	2–5 mg qAM	2–15 mg qAM	• Akathisia • Increased risk of stroke and death in patients with dementia-related psychosis • Parkinsonism
Methylphenidate	2.5–5 mg qAM	2.5–20 mg BID (morning and noon)	• Clear with cardiology or primary care if cardiac risk factors • Weight loss

Behavioral Activation for Older Adults with Depression

Behavioral activation (BA) is a critical and highly effective component of depression treatment. Chances are you are already doing this in some form with your depressed patients. Essentially, BA encourages patients to reengage in their lives and get them moving and feeling better again. This fact sheet will introduce some key features of BA that can be incorporated into short visits, including medication management with add-on psychotherapy.

Basics

- Frequently, individuals experiencing depression stop engaging with friends and activities that bring them happiness. They tell themselves, "I'll restart everything when I feel better." However, setting aside enjoyable pursuits can be counterproductive, leading instead to deepening depression.
- BA is especially relevant for older adults, who may already experience decreased engagement in pleasurable or meaningful activities due to physical or social limitations.
- BA involves identifying activities likely to be rewarding, based on what the patient has previously enjoyed, and setting gradual goals to increase participation in these activities.
- It helps to break the cycle of depression by increasing positive experiences. This improves mood and decreases negative thought patterns.
- For instance, if an older adult has stopped walking in the park due to sadness, a BA approach might involve planning a short walk with a neighbor or family member at first. Breaking down the activity into smaller steps, such as a five-minute stroll, can make it more manageable and easier to initiate.

Implementing Behavioral Activation in Older Adults

Psychoeducation

- Share how BA works and its benefits, emphasizing that reengaging in activities improves mood and reduces depressive symptoms.
- Highlight that actions can improve moods, not just the other way around. This can help shift the patient's perspective on waiting to feel better before doing anything.

Identify interests

- Begin by discussing the older adult's past interests and activities they find enjoyable or meaningful.
- Explore any new interests the older adult might want to pursue.

CASE VIGNETTE: *Mrs. Smith, a 70-year-old widow, mentions she used to enjoy gardening, birdwatching, and attending her local book club but stopped everything once she began feeling depressed.*

Assess current barriers

Understand any physical, psychological, or logistical barriers preventing engagement in activities. Adjustments might be necessary to accommodate limitations.

CASE CONT'D: *Mrs. Smith has arthritis, which limits her gardening, and she no longer drives, affecting her ability to attend the book club.*

Modify existing activities

Work with the older adult to adapt their interests to their current abilities. This might involve creative thinking to modify activities or find accessible alternatives.

CASE CONT'D: *You suggest to Mrs. Smith that using a container garden or a raised bed might minimize bending and kneeling. For birdwatching, suggest she set up a bird feeder visible from a comfortable seat inside or on her patio.*

Introduce new activities

Based on the person's interests and abilities, suggest new activities that have not been considered previously.

CASE CONT'D: *You introduce Mrs. Smith to online book clubs that can be accessed from home, fulfilling her interest in reading and discussion without the need to travel.*

Set gradual goals

Start with small, achievable goals to build confidence and motivation. Gradual progression helps to maintain engagement without overwhelming the individual. Do not force an activity onto an older adult. It should be something they agree to try.

CASE CONT'D: *Mrs. Smith and you begin by setting a goal of spending 15 minutes a day on container gardening or listening to a chapter of an audiobook.*

Schedule activities

Assist the older adult in incorporating activities into their weekly routine to increase the likelihood of follow-through. Encourage them to treat these activities with the same importance as taking a medication.

CASE CONT'D: *You help Mrs. Smith set specific morning gardening times when her energy is highest and schedule book club meetings or reading time in the evening.*

Enhance motivation

- Let the older adult know it is common for people with depression to lose interest in activities they once enjoyed and that it is okay to feel this way.
- Explore ambivalence about reengaging in activities, discussing the pros and cons. Help the patient find their motivation for change.
- Stress that, although it might feel forced at first, taking action despite not feeling like it is a crucial step in breaking the cycle of depression.
- Allow the older adult to choose which activities to start with, giving them control over their recovery process.

Monitor and adjust

- Make it a point to check progress during appointments, discussing what is working and what is not. Be prepared to adjust based on feedback, challenges encountered, and any changes in interests or abilities.
- Document so BA becomes part of the treatment plan and patient instructions.

CASE CONT'D: *Mrs. Smith finds she is enjoying the online book club, so you suggest she increase her frequency of attendance or explore related activities, like writing her own stories.*

Encourage reflection

Discuss the emotions and thoughts associated with engaging in these activities. Reinforce positive experiences to solidify the habit.

CASE CONT'D: *Mrs. Smith shares that gardening makes her feel connected to her late husband, also a gardening enthusiast, bringing her a sense of peace and continuity.*

Positive reinforcement

Celebrate achievements, no matter how small, and encourage the older adult to recognize their progress.

CASE CONT'D: *You recognize the effort it took for Mrs. Smith to adapt to her new gardening setup and applaud her for embracing fresh ways to engage with her interests.*

Cognitive Behavioral Therapy for Older Adults with Depression

Cognitive behavior therapy (CBT) is based on the idea that negative thoughts and unhelpful behaviors contribute to depression and that modifying them can lead to improved symptoms and functioning. CBT is one of the best treatments for depression and is an effective option for older adults (Werson AD et al, *J Affect Disord* 2022;319:189-201). This fact sheet will introduce some key features of CBT that can be incorporated into short visits.

CASE VIGNETTE: *Mrs. Davis is a 68-year-old widow who has been experiencing a noticeable decline in her mood following the passing of her husband last year. A retired schoolteacher, she used to be an active member of her community, often volunteering at her local library and going out with friends. Lately, however, she finds herself withdrawing from these activities, citing a lack of energy and a pervasive sense of sadness. Her grown children have expressed concern about her isolation and encouraged her to seek help. In therapy, she is noted to express a consistent negative outlook, particularly doubting her self-worth.*

Cognitive Restructuring

Definition

Cognitive restructuring aims to *identify*, *challenge*, and *modify* thoughts that add to depression.

Identify negative thoughts

Often these are recurring beliefs and take the form of absolutes and overgeneralizations.

- Pay attention to the following themes, referred to as "Beck's Cognitive Triad of Depression":
  - I'm deficient.
  - The world is a hostile place.
  - Things will never get better.
- Some examples are:
  - "My life has been a waste."
  - "I'm a burden to my family and friends."
  - "No one wants to spend time with me."
  - "It's pointless to try anything new at my age."

Challenge the thoughts

- Once negative views are identified, help patients recognize their distorted thinking by pointing out overgeneralizations, all-or-nothing thinking, or other errors in logic.
- Next, ask patients to examine the evidence for and against their beliefs.
- For example, Mrs. Davis thinks, "My friends don't want to spend time with me because I'm not fun anymore." Ask Mrs. Davis:
  - What facts support this statement?
    - "Can you think of specific instances where your friends explicitly said they didn't want to spend time with you because they didn't find you fun?"
  - Is there evidence to the contrary?
    - "Have there been occasions when your friends reached out to spend time with you or enjoyed your company? What about times when you felt connected and had a good time together?"
    - "Have you had other experiences recently where you had fun with people?"
    - "Could you be jumping to conclusions?"
  - What would you tell a friend with the same thought?
    - "If a friend came to you feeling this way, saying they believe they're no longer fun and that's why people don't want to spend time with them, what would you tell them? Would you agree with their assessment, or might you challenge their perception based on what you know about them?"
  - What would a friend say about your thought?
    - "Imagine you shared this thought with one of your friends. What do you think they would say? Do you think they might offer examples of times you've been fun to be around, or might they express appreciation for your qualities beyond just being 'fun'?"

Modify or reframe the thought

- Work together, using the "Challenge the Thought" discussion, to develop a more balanced and nuanced statement. Have the patient say the reframed thought out loud.

- For example, for Mrs. Davis, a reworked thought could be, "Everyone has moments when they feel more or less fun. Friends understand this. Instead of assuming they don't want to spend time with me, I can tell them how I feel and explore new ways to enjoy our time together, embracing our current interests and life stages. My friends also might be dealing with their own issues right now, which might limit their enjoyment of activities."

Resources

CBT self-help books on depression

Feeling Good: The New Mood Therapy by David D. Burns: Offers insights into CBT techniques and practical strategies for overcoming depression.

Online resources

- *Get Self Help* (https://tinyurl.com/pksatfr4): Offers CBT self-help and therapy resources, including a variety of free worksheets on cognitive distortions, thought records, and behavioral activation techniques. The site also offers guides and examples on effectively using the worksheets.
- *MoodGYM* (moodgym.com.au): An interactive web program designed to prevent and decrease symptoms of depression through cognitive behavioral exercises.
- *Psychology Tools* (psychologytools.com): Offers a wide range of CBT worksheets, handouts, and resources. These include detailed reports for identifying and challenging cognitive distortions, guides for completing thought change records, and plans for behavioral activation. Many resources are free, with more comprehensive tools accessible through a paid subscription.
- *Therapist Aid* (therapistaid.com): Provides free therapy worksheets, tools, and handouts for mental health professionals and individuals. There are worksheets on cognitive distortions, activities aimed at behavioral activation, and templates for thought records. Free, with the option for more resources through a paid subscription.

Interpersonal Therapy in Late-Life Depression

Interpersonal Therapy (IPT) is based on the idea that distressing personal relationships and life events contribute to depression. While mainly studied in adults, it may be helpful for older adults because late life often involves confronting the core issues that IPT addresses. These include conflicts with others, changing life roles, grief, and difficulties in keeping/maintaining relationships. IPT empowers patients to improve their communication skills and strengthen social connections. While IPT is typically delivered over 12 to 16 sessions by a trained therapist, this fact sheet will introduce some key features that can be incorporated into brief visits.

Interpersonal Assessment

For an older adult with depression, use targeted questions to quickly identify the primary problem area:

- "Have there been any significant changes in your life recently?"
- "Do you find yourself in conflict with friends or family?"
- "Have you been dealing with feelings of loss?"

Identification of specific problem areas

- *Grief:* Inquire about recent losses and the patient's process of mourning. Distinguish between normal grief and complicated grief, where the intensity of grief is prolonged and interferes with functioning.
- *Interpersonal deficits:* Explore the patient's ability to initiate and maintain close relationships. Identify patterns of isolation, withdrawal, or chronic conflicts in relationships.
- *Role disputes:* Pinpoint any ongoing conflicts with significant others that may be contributing to the patient's depression. Explore the nature of these disputes, the roles involved, and the patient's feelings and behaviors in these conflicts.
- *Role transitions:* Discuss any recent or impending changes in life roles, such as retirement, relocation, changes in health status, or loss of a significant relationship.

Areas of Intervention

Grief

CASE VIGNETTE 1: *Mr. Silva, an 80-year-old widower, is grieving the loss of his wife. An IPT approach to support him could involve providing space to express his feelings, share memories, and explore the impact of his loss. Possible strategies might include starting a meaningful project to honor his wife's memory and encouraging a gradual re-engagement in social activities.*

- *Definition:* Grief is the process of experiencing psychological, social, and physical reactions to the perception of loss.
- *Relevance:* Older adults often face multiple losses, including the deaths of loved ones, loss of independence, or loss of physical health.
- *Goals*
  - Facilitate the expression of grief and mourning.
    - Create a safe space for patients to talk about their feelings.
    - Suggest writing letters to the deceased or journaling about feelings.
    - Art or writing can help express emotions that might be difficult to articulate.
  - Help the patient adjust to life without the deceased or to what was lost.
    - Discuss establishing new daily routines that do not include the loss.
  - Reinforce healthy memories and connections.
    - Help the patient create a memory box or a scrapbook filled with photos, letters, and other mementos that celebrate the deceased's life.
    - Encourage sharing stories about the loved one with friends or family, or within a support group, to keep the person's memory alive and meaningful.
  - Gradually encourage activities that were previously enjoyed.
    - Slowly reintroduce activities the patient used to enjoy. Recommend that the patient initially participate in these activities with a supportive friend or family member.
  - Develop new relationships.
    - Encourage joining clubs or senior groups aligned with the patient's interests (eg, book clubs, religious organizations, walking groups) to facilitate opportunities for new friendships.
  - Address any guilt or anger.

- *Sample discussion questions*
  - "Can you tell me about the person you've lost?"
  - "What do you miss most about them?"
  - "Are there things you feel were left unsaid or unfinished?"
  - "How has your life changed since their passing?"
  - "What emotions do you experience when you think about them now?"

Interpersonal deficits

CASE VIGNETTE 2: *Mrs. Lin, a 75-year-old woman, is experiencing loneliness after the deaths of many close friends. An IPT approach would help her address fears about making new connections, explore interests that could lead to social interactions, and practice conversational skills. An action plan might be to join a senior center and reconnect with family members.*

- *Definition:* Social deficits may become an issue for patients with a history of difficulty forming and maintaining relationships. These may become more pronounced in later life due to the loss of existing social contacts.
- *Relevance:* Deficits could lead to social isolation and lack of support, contributing to depression.
- *Therapy goals*
  - Enhance social skills.
    - Focus on specific skills, such as initiating conversations, maintaining eye contact, listening actively, and understanding nonverbal cues.
    - Role-playing exercises can help people build conversational skills, handle social cues, and respond to different social situations.
  - Increase opportunities for social interactions.
    - Encourage participation in community events or activities that align with the individual's interests. This could include joining clubs, attending local events, participating in workshops, or attending the local senior center.
    - Suggest volunteer opportunities to meet new people.
  - Develop new relationships or strengthen existing ones.
    - Work with the individual to set specific, achievable goals for developing new relationships and deepening existing ones. For instance, you might suggest that they initiate one new conversation per week or invite a friend over for coffee.
    - Encourage regular follow-ups: To maintain relationships, recommend frequently reaching out to contacts. Suggest scheduling regular calls and meetings.
    - Encourage older adults to join groups (eg, book clubs, gardening clubs, craft groups) where they can meet others with similar interests.
- *Sample discussion questions*
  - "Do you find it difficult to make or keep friends? Can you tell me more about that?"
  - "What do you think holds you back in your relationships?"
  - "How do you usually feel in social situations?"
  - "Can you describe a recent interaction that didn't go as well as you'd hoped?"
  - "What qualities do you look for in a friend or companion?"

Role disputes

Case Vignette 3: *Mr. Tyson, a 70-year-old man, does not agree with his son's recommendation to move to an assisted living facility. Possible IPT approaches to the dispute include identifying the communication breakdown, facilitating a family meeting to discuss each party's concerns, and exploring compromise positions. A reasonable outcome might be improved mutual understanding and a trial agreement for in-home care with regular evaluations.*

- *Definition:* Conflicts arise when the patient and others have differing expectations about their relationship.
- *Relevance:* Older adults may face disputes with adult children, caregivers, or spouses, particularly regarding autonomy, care needs, and lifestyle choices.
- *Goals*
  - Identify the nature of the dispute.
    - Encourage both parties involved to practice active listening.

    - Use clarifying questions to ensure that each person understands the other's perspective.
  - Communicate feelings and needs effectively.
    - Teach the use of "I" statements to express feelings and needs without blaming the other person. For example, instead of saying, "You aren't listening to me," which blames the other person and makes an assumption about them, say, "I feel like we aren't communicating clearly." This opens the door for a more empathetic response and constructive dialogue rather than a defensive or hostile exchange.
    - Encourage each person to consider the other's feelings and viewpoints.
  - Negotiate a new understanding or solution.
    - Facilitate having everyone suggest solutions to the conflict without criticism.
- *Sample discussion questions*
  - "Can you describe a recent argument or disagreement with [the person]?"
  - "What do you think [the person] expects from you in this relationship?"
  - "How do your expectations of the relationship differ from theirs?"
  - "What was your relationship like before the problem started?"
  - "How have you tried to resolve these disputes? What was the outcome?"

Role transitions

CASE VIGNETTE 4: *Ms. Jackson, a 65-year-old woman, is struggling with retirement and loss of professional identity. An IPT approach might be to help her grieve the loss of her career, explore aspects of her identity beyond work, and identify new roles and activities. One outcome could be volunteering in a hospital, leading to increased social engagement.*

- *Definition:* Older adults face significant life changes, such as retirement, loss of independence, or becoming a caregiver, all of which can contribute to depression.
- *Relevance:* Such transitions can challenge an older adult's sense of identity and purpose.
- *Therapy goals*
  - Mourn the loss of the old role.
    - Allow individuals to express their feelings about losing their previous role.
    - Validate feelings of sadness or frustration.
  - Explore the positive and negative aspects of the new role.
    - The new role might be a combination of many things—grandparent, volunteer, hobbyist, friend, or student.
    - Help the individual list the advantages and disadvantages of their new role. This can help them provide a balanced view and process the transition more effectively.
    - Encourage exploration of what the new role entails. This could involve discussing potential opportunities and challenges, setting short-term goals, and identifying necessary resources for the change.
    - Identify others who have thrived in their new roles, eg, in retirement. Learning how others have coped can provide inspiration and strategies.
  - Improve satisfaction with the new role.
    - Help set achievable expectations for the new role.
    - Encourage connecting to supports to help with the transition.
- *Sample discussion questions*
  - "What has been the hardest part of the transition away from [the role] for you?"
  - "How do you feel about leaving behind being [the role]?"
  - "What changes are you finding challenging?"
  - "Can you think of any positive aspects or opportunities in this [new role]?"

Online Resources and Websites

Therapist Aid

- *URLs:* https://tinyurl.com/59fu8hdd *and* https://tinyurl.com/39rktwx8
- *Offers many free and easy-to-use worksheets on:*
  - Active listening
  - Assertive communication
  - Communications skills
  - "I" statements
  - Relationship conflict resolution
  - Ways to build social support

COMMON LATE-LIFE PSYCHIATRIC DISORDERS

Insomnia

Insomnia in Older Adults: Nonpharmacological Treatment

Insomnia is subjective discontent with sleep quality or quantity. As many as 50% of older adults report sleep difficulties, while the prevalence of insomnia disorder ranges from 12%–20% (Patel D et al, *J Clin Sleep Med* 2018;14(6):1017–1024). This fact sheet will discuss nonpharmacological management of insomnia in older adults.

What Is Insomnia?

- There are two types of insomnia
  - Difficulty initiating sleep (sleep-onset insomnia)
  - Frequent awakenings or early-morning awakening (sleep-maintenance insomnia)
- Insomnia is classified as
  - Episodic (1 to <3 months)
  - Persistent (≥3 nights per week for >3 months)
  - Recurrent (≥2 episodes/year)

How to Decide Whether to Use Medication vs Nonmedication Approaches

I will start with nonmedication approaches in the following circumstances:

- The patient prefers to avoid medication.
- Medication options would not be safe due to high fall risk, cognitive impairment, or other factors.
- The insomnia is mild to moderate in severity.
- There is a clear behavioral or environmental cause that can be addressed.

Nonpharmacologic Approaches

The following approaches include some that you can do in the office with patients and others that you may need to refer to a specialized therapist, if one is available.

Sleep hygiene

- Maintain regular sleep/wake times.
- Exercise in the morning or afternoon.
- Optimize bedroom environment (dark, quiet, and cool).
- Reduce stimulants like caffeine and nicotine from lunch onward.
- Reduce ambient noise at night. Consider masking noise with soft music or a sound machine.
- Block outside light at night with black-out curtains.
- Limit daytime napping and fluids before bedtime.
- Avoid alcohol, which can cause fragmented sleep.

Cognitive behavioral therapy for insomnia (CBT-I)

- *Description:* Gold-standard treatment for insomnia; consists of 6 to 10 sessions. CBT-I is a straightforward therapy to learn, otherwise consider referring to a therapist trained in CBT-I who has experience working with older adults.
- *Efficacy:* Randomized controlled trials in older adults have shown that CBT-I is more effective and has longer-lasting therapeutic effects than pharmacological treatments (Flaxer JM et al, *Am J Geriatr Psychiatry* 2021;29(6):585-603).
- *Components*
  - Sleep hygiene education
  - Sleep restriction therapy
    - Starting point: Patients begin by restricting their time in bed to match their average total sleep time, estimated from a two-week sleep diary.
    - Calculate sleep efficiency: Sleep efficiency is estimated as the percentage of time spent asleep out of the total time in bed.
    - Adjustments based on efficiency:
      - If sleep efficiency is >90% (indicating most of the time in bed is spent asleep), increase the total sleep time by 15 minutes.
      - If sleep efficiency is <85% (indicating too much time is spent awake), reduce total sleep time by 15 minutes.
    - Goal: These adjustments help determine the optimal amount of sleep needed while ensuring that most of the time in bed is spent sleeping (Suzuki K et al, *J Gen Fam Med* 2017;18(2):61–71).
  - Stimulus control therapy: Counsel patients to go to bed only when sleepy and to use the bed only for sleep or sex. If the patient is unable to fall asleep for 20 minutes, they should get out of bed and do something nonstimulating until sleepy again. The goal is to create an association between the bed and sleep rather than between the bed and wakefulness or frustration.

Brief behavioral treatment for chronic insomnia (BBTI)

- *Description:* Shorter, four-session version of CBT-I.
- *Efficacy:* Effective in older adults, with benefits lasting six months and beyond (Buysse DJ et al, *Arch Intern Med* 2011;171(10):887–895).

Relaxation techniques prior to bedtime

- Progressive muscle relaxation.
- Guided imagery.
- Mindfulness and diaphragmatic breathing.
- Yoga and meditation.
- See "Anxiety-Reduction Techniques: Cognitive Restructuring and Relaxation in Older Adults" [page 30] fact sheet in the "Anxiety Disorders" section of this book.

Bright light therapy

- *Use:* Helps to strengthen circadian rhythms and establish a healthy sleep-wake cycle.
- *Efficacy:* May have a favorable effect in older adults.
- *Implementation:* Provide white light sources with a bluish tint that have at least 1,000 lux during daytime hours, on mornings after awakening, or when the patient becomes more tired outside of regular sleeping times (Brewster G et al, *Sleep Med Clin* 2018;13(1):13–19).

Other interventions

- *Acupuncture:* Specific points on the body are stimulated by inserting thin needles through the skin. It has been shown to be effective in improving insomnia in older adults.
- *Chamomile tea*
- *Lavender oil*
- *Music therapy*

Mobile apps

- *CBT-I coach*
- *YouTube*: Provides access to a variety of free sleep music, sounds, and meditation videos.

Nonpharmacologic Approaches for Specific Sleep Disorders

Sleep apnea

Refer for polysomnography and consider continuous positive airway pressure therapy. A sleep specialist or pulmonologist will be best suited to manage sleep apnea.

Restless legs syndrome and periodic limb movement disorder

- Recommend iron supplements if ferritin is low.
- Eliminate or reduce caffeine and serotonergic antidepressants.
- Beneficial evening treatments include warm baths, lower extremity massages (some people use massagers), warming packs, relaxation techniques, and stretching.
- Suggest regular moderate exercise, totaling at least 2.5 hours a week.

Insomnia in Older Adults: Medication Treatment

Insomnia presents unique treatment challenges in older adults due to the potential for adverse drug reactions. This fact sheet offers an overview of pharmacological options, including FDA-approved medications, off-label uses for comorbid conditions, and over-the-counter (OTC) remedies, emphasizing considerations for older adults.

FDA-Approved Medications for Insomnia (In Order of Preference)

Ramelteon (Rozerem)

- *Dose:* 8 mg at bedtime
- *Indications:* Sleep-onset insomnia, delayed sleep phase syndrome
- *Side effects:* Somnolence, headache, dizziness
- *Considerations:* Minimal risk of dependency; well-suited for long-term use.

Doxepin (Silenor)

- *Dose:* 3–6 mg at bedtime
- *Indications:* Sleep-maintenance insomnia
- *Side effects:* Nausea, somnolence, dizziness, constipation, dry mouth
- *Considerations:* Avoid in patients with narrow-angle glaucoma, urinary retention, or sleep apnea due to its anticholinergic effects.

Lemborexant (Dayvigo)

- *Dose:* 5–10 mg at bedtime
- *Indications:* Sleep-onset and maintenance insomnia
- *Side effects:* Somnolence, headache, abnormal dreams, sleep paralysis
- *Considerations:*
  - Potential for next-day somnolence, especially at the 10 mg dose. It is contraindicated with strong CYP3A4 inhibitors. Avoid in patients with narcolepsy.
  - In people over 65, lemborexant does not impair memory, affect ability to awaken to nighttime noises, impact tests of memory and attention, or impair next-day driving performance (Gotfried MH et al, *Drugs Aging* 2024;41(9):741-752).

Suvorexant (Belsomra)

- *Dose:* 5–20 mg at bedtime
- *Indications:* Sleep-onset and maintenance insomnia
- *Side effects:* Somnolence, headache, dizziness, abnormal dreams, dry mouth, sleep paralysis
- *Considerations:* Monitor for next-day somnolence. It is contraindicated with strong CYP3A4 inhibitors. Avoid in patients with narcolepsy.

Off-Label Medications for Insomnia

- *Gabapentin:* Effective for insomnia; FDA-approved for neuropathic pain and restless legs syndrome, used in doses of 100–400 mg at bedtime.
- *Mirtazapine:* Suitable for patients with depression; initiates sleep at doses of 7.5–15 mg.
- *Quetiapine:* May be used for insomnia associated with psychosis or bipolar disorder, with careful monitoring for metabolic side effects.
- *Trazodone:* Not recommended for the primary treatment of sleep onset or maintenance issues, but it can help with insomnia occurring in the context of depression.

OTC Options

- *Melatonin:* Can aid in sleep initiation; doses of 0.5–6 mg are mildly helpful; give 3 hours prior to bedtime. Time release forms may help those who wake up during the night and are unable to return to sleep.
- *Valerian root:* Some evidence suggests it may improve sleep quality; start with 600 mg qHS.

Riskier Medications

- *Benzodiazepines (BZD) and Z-drugs (eg, zaleplon, zolpidem)*
  - Avoid prescribing in older adults due to potential side effects (delirium, falls, withdrawal; complex sleep-related behaviors, like sleepwalking, sleep talking, nocturnal eating, hallucinations, and confused arousals).
  - BZDs are uniquely effective for some patients when other treatments have failed or when the patient has taken BZDs for decades. Such patients may be very reluctant to taper off them. An individualized approach is necessary here, taking into account the variability of individual responses after conducting a thorough risk-benefit analysis.

Sometimes tapering off long-standing BZDs can result in significant worsening of symptoms and functional decline.

- If continuation or initiation of BZDs or Z-drugs is deemed necessary, use the lowest effective dose and shorter-acting agents, such as temazepam or lorazepam to minimize adverse effects. Enact regular monitoring and reevaluation of the treatment plan to ensure patient safety.

- *OTC Medications*
  - Many OTC agents (eg, diphenhydramine and doxylamine), have significant anticholinergic activity. Warn older adults to avoid them due to risk of increased confusion.

COMMON LATE-LIFE PSYCHIATRIC DISORDERS

Personality Disorders

Personality Disorders in Older Adults

Personality disorders (PDs) in older adults are understudied and underdiagnosed. The most common PDs in older adults, in order of prevalence, are obsessive-compulsive, paranoid, narcissistic, and avoidant.

CASE VIGNETTE: *Mr. Ewing, an 82-year-old retired accountant, is brought to the clinic by his son for conflicts at home. He insists every household item must be kept in a precise location, checks locks repeatedly, and berates his son for minor deviations in daily routines. These behaviors have intensified since his wife passed away six months ago. The clinical picture is suggestive of OCPD exacerbated by bereavement, now causing significant caregiver strain.*

Clinical Features in Older Adults

- *Age-related changes:* Life transitions (retirement, bereavement, health decline) can exacerbate maladaptive personality traits as older adults lose independence and rely more on others.
- *Cognitive vs. personality changes:* Older adults with PDs may develop increased suspiciousness or rigidity, which can mask underlying cognitive decline.
- *Decline in impulsivity*: People with borderline PD show fewer self-harming acts and less impulsivity in later life but fear of abandonment and poor interpersonal functioning persist. Antisocial behavior including impulsive actions and legal trouble decreases in older age.
- *Increased interpersonal strain*: Family or caregiver relationships can become tense, especially if the older adult requires more assistance but resists due to untrusting or obsessive traits.

Table 11: **Personality Disorders in Older vs Younger Adults**

Aspect	Older Adults	Younger Adults
Prevalence	11%–15% in the community; 58% in nursing homes	9%–13% in the general population
Onset	Longstanding patterns become more apparent under stress (eg, bereavement, retirement)	Typically identified in late adolescence or early adulthood
Common Types	Obsessive-compulsive, paranoid, narcissistic, avoidant	Borderline, antisocial, narcissistic
Clinical Features	More likely to be: male, married, have mixed PDs, high polypharmacy	More frequent: impulsivity, self-harm, chronic unstable relationships
Impulsivity	Tends to decrease with age, though core emotional dysregulation (eg, fear of abandonment) may persist	Often high (eg, reckless behavior, self-injury)
Interpersonal Conflicts	May shift to strained caregiver/family relationships, sometimes leading to isolation	Usually with peers or significant others
Rigidity/Suspiciousness	Can intensify due to medical issues, reliance on caregivers, fear of vulnerability	May be present but less tied to health concerns
Cognitive Overlay	Need to rule out dementia or delirium; suspiciousness or rigidity may mask cognitive decline	Typically, intact cognitive functioning

Source: Penders KAP et al, *Curr Psychiatry Rep 2020*;22(3):14; Treagust N et al, *Int J Geriatr Psychiatry* 2022;37(12):10.1002/gps.5837.

Treatment Approaches (Few Studies Exist)

Psychotherapy (cornerstone treatment)

- *Dialectical Behavior Therapy (DBT)*
  - DBT focuses on helping patients develop skills in mindfulness, distress tolerance, emotional regulation, and interpersonal effectiveness.
  - It is used for patients with borderline PD but is also effective for comorbid PD and depression.
  - Modules can be modified for slower pacing in older adults.

- *Schema Therapy*
  - Addresses longstanding cognitive and emotional patterns ("maladaptive schemas"). It focuses on identifying and modifying maladaptive schemas.
  - It can be tailored to older adults by incorporating life review, simplified imagery rescripting, and compassion-focused techniques.
  - It is effective for older adults with cluster C PDs or another specified PD with cluster C traits (Penders KAP et al, *Curr Psychiatry Rep* 2020).
- *Systems Training for Emotional Predictability and Problem-Solving (STEPPS):*
  - This cognitive behavioral therapy-based group treatment has shown feasibility in older adults, particularly for those with borderline PD, improving emotion regulation and self-control (Ekiz E et al, *Behav Cogn Psychother* 2023;51(1):105-109).
- *Cognitive Behavioral Therapy (CBT):*
  - Targets maladaptive thoughts and behaviors; it can be adapted for sensory or mobility limitations.

Pharmacotherapy (for management of comorbid conditions or specific symptoms)

- *Antidepressants, such as selective serotonin reuptake inhibitors (SSRIs)*: Can help manage co-occurring depression, anxiety, or obsessional thinking.
- *Low-dose antipsychotics*: May assist with extreme suspiciousness in people with paranoid PD or with aggression, anger, impulsivity, or mood lability in people with other PDs. Use cautiously due to their side effect profile (eg, extrapyramidal symptoms, metabolic syndrome, sedation).
- *Mood stabilizers*: Lamotrigine may improve impulse control and affective instability in people with borderline PD.

Practical tips for clinicians

- *Take a long view*: Inquire about longstanding interpersonal patterns, personality traits, and past stressors or traumas.
- *Rule out other causes*: Assess for dementia, delirium, or other medical conditions mimicking personality changes.
- *Build therapeutic alliance*: Older adults with paranoid or rigid traits may require extra time to establish trust.
- *Focus on function*: Emphasize practical strategies (eg, daily routines) that support autonomy and health adherence.
- *Involve caregivers*: Provide psychoeducation to family members, ensuring they understand the chronic nature of PDs, including that complete "personality change" is unlikely; however, symptom reduction and improved adaptive functioning are achievable goals with consistent intervention.

Challenging Situations with Older Adults

Older adults may exhibit a range of challenging personality traits that can stem from cognitive decline, psychiatric disorders, medical illnesses, daily life stresses, or loss of independence. Core principles to manage them are remaining patient and empathic, discussing instead of commanding, offering choices when possible, and setting clear consequences (https://tinyurl.com/ncuzxtca). This fact sheet will review some common manifestations of puzzling personality traits in older adults and ways to address them.

CASE VIGNETTE 1: *Mr. Cohen, a 65-year-old patient with depression, resists starting a prescribed exercise regimen.*

Rigidity

May manifest as unwillingness to adapt to new routines, plans, or recommendations.

Tips

- Validate the older adult's feelings and acknowledge the difficulty of changing.
- Connect new routines to personal goals or interests.
  - For example, Mr. Cohen may want to stay active enough to play with his grandchildren. He could be encouraged to follow an exercise routine emphasizing walking and strength training to meet this goal, thereby linking exercise to his desire of playing with his grandkids.
- Introduce changes incrementally and only with the patient's buy-in.

Discussion questions

- "Can you tell me more about why you don't want to do the exercises?"
- "Do you think you'll get any benefit from them?"
- "How can we change the exercises so they feel more doable for you?"
- "How can we help you get started?"

CASE VIGNETTE 2: *Ms. Petrov, a 74-year-old patient, demands meals and medications at times that disrupt the established routine of her care facility.*

Excessive or Unreasonable Requests or Expectations

Examples

- Demanding constant attention from staff or caregivers.
- Requesting frequent or unnecessary medical tests or procedures.
- Insisting on specific medications (eg, alprazolam for generalized anxiety disorder rather than a selective serotonin reuptake inhibitor).
- Demanding special treatment (eg, for nursing staff to administer bedtime medications at precisely 10 pm).

Tips

- Maintain a calm, professional demeanor.
- Set clear boundaries and explain the rationale behind policies.
- Avoid arguing or trying to reason, as this can increase resistance.
- Offer alternatives that align with what is feasible within the care setting.
- Educate regarding the roles and availability of staff to meet demands.
- Suggest the patient discuss their concerns with the patient advocate if they remain dissatisfied. This recommendation conveys the message that there is "nothing to hide."

Discussion questions

- "What's important to you about having meals and medications at these specific times?"
- "Can we explore other ways to accommodate your needs that also fit within our schedule?"
- "Is there a compromise that would make you feel heard and keep our unit running smoothly?"

CASE VIGNETTE 3: *Mrs. Anderson, a 77-year-old patient, frequently visits the hospital, reporting varied and unspecific symptoms like stomach aches and headaches. Medical testing is consistently unremarkable and there is no apparent cause.*

Dealing with Somatic Preoccupation

Somatic preoccupation refers to patients excessively focused on physical symptoms, which may or may not have a discernible medical basis. Such patients often require a lot of reassurance and can stress staff resources.

Discussion points

- Validate the symptoms as real and distressing.
  - "I can see how much these symptoms are bothering you, and it's important that we take them seriously."
- Discourage excessive medical testing, which can reinforce the belief that a serious illness is being missed and may actually worsen health anxiety.
  - I will usually say, "I have great news. You've had a lot of tests done, and if there was a major issue like cancer, a stroke, or a heart attack, the doctors would've found it. There are probably a lot of different things going on right now that are contributing to how you're feeling. That's why they sent me (a consultant) to help figure it out."
- Discuss the multifactorial nature of their symptoms. Explain that symptoms can have complex causes that may involve other factors.
  - "While we haven't found a medical illness that explains your symptoms, this doesn't mean the symptoms aren't real. Factors like stress, lifestyle, and thinking can significantly influence how we feel physically."
- Explain the mind-body connection.
  - "Emotions and physical health are deeply interconnected. Stress, anxiety, or other struggles can activate the body's stress response, leading to physical symptoms."
- Recommend a holistic approach to treatment that includes psychological and physical health.
  - "Managing these symptoms will require a holistic approach. How do you feel about exploring some options that might include both physical and mental health care?"
- Shift the focus from symptoms to improving quality of life and functionality.
  - "Let's work on strategies to help you manage your symptoms so they interfere less with your daily life. For example, what activities have you stopped doing that you'd like to start again?"
- Establish regular follow-up or consultations in the hospital to monitor the patient's symptoms and modify the treatment plan, as needed.

CASE VIGNETTE 4: *Mr. Morales, a 68-year-old patient, repeatedly requests alprazolam and is reluctant to try psychotherapy or other anxiety-reduction techniques.*

Managing Medication-Focused Patients

Discussion points

- Establish a strong therapeutic relationship through empathy, active listening, and regular follow-ups.
- An excessive focus on medications can be a symptom of underlying anxieties, fears, or misinformation. Uncover and address these root causes.
- Enforce policies regarding prescription practices firmly but kindly.
- Clearly explain how medications work, their potential side effects, and why certain medications may not be suitable or necessary.
  - "There are risks when benzodiazepines are prescribed to older patients. Would you like to discuss them?"
- Highlight the benefits of a comprehensive treatment approach that includes lifestyle modifications and nonpharmacological treatments.
  - "It's important for us to use all the tools we have, not just medications."
- Introduce and discuss alternative therapies such as physical therapy, psychotherapy, and exercise programs, explaining how these can complement or sometimes substitute for medications.
  - "Can we explore what concerns you have about psychotherapy? I've found it very effective for others with similar complaints."

CASE VIGNETTE 5: *Mr. Mensah, a 71-year-old patient, is ready for discharge from the inpatient psychiatric unit. He expresses reluctance to leave because he feels safe in the hospital and likes the staff.*

Handling Patients Nervous about Discharge

Discussion points

- Patients may resist discharge due to fear, uncertainty, or dissatisfaction with their progress. Recognize and validate the patient's emotions about discharge.
  - "It can be scary to leave, especially when you've done so well here and aren't sure how things will be back at home. Do you have specific concerns about leaving the hospital?"
- Directly address any apprehensions the patient has about leaving. This could include worries about managing their illness, lack of support at home, or uncertainty about follow-up care.
  - "What aspects of being here make you feel safe? What strengths do you feel you've developed during your treatment that you can rely on moving forward? Understanding this can help us ensure you feel secure even after discharge."
- For issues related to lack of housing, social support, or financial resources, patients may benefit from referral to case management, community outreach organizations, advocacy groups, or legal aid services.
  - "What can we add to your discharge plan to make you feel more supported once you leave?"
- During the hospitalization, encourage greater involvement from the patient's family, friends, or community resources. A strong support network can offer emotional comfort and practical assistance after discharge. Arrange a meeting with the patient and their family before discharge to ensure everyone understands the plan.
  - "Who will support you after you leave the hospital? Let's talk about how you can communicate your needs and concerns with them."
  - "There are also community resources available, like your town's senior center. Would you like more information about them?"
- Before discharge, ensure that the patient has a robust plan in place. This may involve setting up outpatient programs/appointments or arranging in-home services if available.
  - "Let's review your follow-up care plan together. We've coordinated for you to start treatment in the geriatric day program, which includes support from a team of psychiatrists, psychologists, social workers, therapists, and nurses. You'll attend five days a week, Monday through Friday. How do you feel about this plan?"

COMMON LATE-LIFE PSYCHIATRIC DISORDERS

Schizophrenia and Other Psychotic Disorders

Psychosis in Older Adults: Diagnosis and Treatment

Schizophrenia spectrum disorders and other manifestations of psychosis in older adults have different presentations and treatment considerations compared to younger individuals. The following is an overview of these variances and practical approaches for clinicians.

Epidemiology

- *Prevalence:* While the prevalence of psychotic symptoms increases with age, particularly in those with dementia or depression, schizophrenia affects a smaller subset of older adults, comprising about 0.5%, compared to 1% of adults.
- *Age of onset:* Schizophrenia typically starts in late adolescence or early adulthood, but a large portion of patients experience late-onset (after age 40) or very late-onset (after age 60) schizophrenia.

Differences in Presentation of Psychosis in Older Versus Younger Adults

Cognitive decline: Psychotic symptoms frequently emerge in the context of established cognitive impairments such as dementia or delirium.

Nature of psychotic symptoms

- *Delusions:* More likely to consist of persecutory or somatic beliefs.
- *Hallucinations:* Visual hallucinations are more common in older adults, especially when due to delirium or dementia; auditory hallucinations are more prevalent in younger individuals.

Comorbid conditions

- Older adults have a higher prevalence of medical illnesses or medications (eg, Parkinson's disease and dopamine agonist prescriptions), which can contribute to psychosis.
- Increased sensitivity to medication side effects and higher risk of polypharmacy should influence medication selection.

Functional impact

Psychotic disorders result in a greater impact on daily functioning and a higher risk of hospitalization or institutionalization.

Clinical Presentations

Schizoaffective disorder

- *Description:* While schizoaffective disorder has a better prognosis in younger adults than schizophrenia, in older adults, it may be more severe, more complex to treat, and linked with a higher rate of dying by suicide. Older adults with schizoaffective disorder bear close monitoring (Post F, *Br J Psychiat* 1971;118(545):437-445).
- *Symptoms:* Composed of features of both schizophrenia and a mood disorder (either bipolar or depressive type).

Late-onset schizophrenia (LOS)

- *Epidemiology:* 20%–25% of patients with schizophrenia experience the onset of the disorder after age 40, with a greater proportion being women (Reinhardt MM and Cohen CL, *Curr Psychiatry Rep* 2015;17(2):1).
- *Symptoms:* Like early-onset schizophrenia (EOS), symptoms consist predominantly of paranoia and auditory hallucinations, with relatively preserved cognitive function. Patients with LOS have fewer negative symptoms.
- *Course:* Typically, less severe than EOS, with a better prognosis and response to lower doses of antipsychotics.

Very late-onset schizophrenia-like psychosis (VLOSLP)

- *Description:* People with VLOSLP have more brain abnormalities and neuropsychological deficits than people with other forms of schizophrenia, indicating a potential neurodegenerative origin. Many more women have VLOSLP and often there is less family history of schizophrenia (Reinhardt MM and Cohen CL, *Curr Psychiatry Rep* 2015).
- *Symptoms:* There is a greater frequency of persecutory delusions and hallucinations—visual, tactile, and olfactory. VLOSLP is not associated with negative symptoms or formal thought disorder (Reinhardt MM and Cohen CL, *Curr Psychiatry Rep* 2015).
- *Course:* It is often associated with sensory deficits (eg, hearing or vision loss) and cerebrovascular disease.

Delusional disorder (DD)

- *Epidemiology:* Reports show an occurrence of 0.03 % in older adults, with women marginally more affected than men (Meesters PD et al, *Am J Geriatr Psychiatry* 2012;20(1):18-28).
- *Symptoms:* Patients have persistent delusions without prominent hallucinations. Common themes include persecution, jealousy, and somatic concerns.
- *Course:* Onset is typically in middle or late adulthood. DD has a chronic course but less severe functional impairment compared to schizophrenia. In older adults, hearing and visual abnormalities might play a role in its development, so recommend to have them checked.

Table 12: **Differential Diagnosis of Psychosis in Older Adults***

#	Differential Diagnosis	Onset and Timing	Presenting Symptoms	Treatment Approach	Prognosis
1	**Psychotic Disorder due to Another Medical Condition** (eg, electrolyte imbalances— hyponatremia, hypercalcemia, hyperthyroidism, hypothyroidism, vitamin B12 deficiency)	Variable, often sudden	Depends on specific illness (eg, infections, metabolic disturbances)	Treat underlying cause, order second-generation antipsychotics if symptoms threaten safety or significantly impair functioning, provide supportive care	Reversible with treatment, risk of recurrence
2	**Substance-Induced Psychotic Disorders** (eg, alcohol intoxication or withdrawal; cannabis intoxication; prescription medications such as anticholinergics, dopaminergics, sedatives, and steroids; illicit drugs such as cocaine, methamphetamines, and PCP)	Variable, often sudden	Depends on specific substance	Discontinue offending substance, order second-generation antipsychotics if symptoms threaten safety or significantly impair functioning, offer alcohol or drug rehabilitation, provide supportive care	Reversible with treatment, risk of recurrence
3	**Delirium**	Acute, hours to days	Agitation, confusion, perceptual disturbances	Treat underlying cause, use antipsychotics for dangerous or threatening behaviors	Often reversible with treatment
4	**Dementia**	Gradual, months to years	Cognitive decline with neuropsychiatric symptoms	Cognitive enhancers, order second-generation antipsychotics (SGAs) if symptoms threaten safety or cause significant distress, increased risk of stroke and death when antipsychotics used to treat "dementia-related psychosis," incorporate nonpharmacological treatments.	Progressive, varies by type
5	**Major Depressive Disorder with Psychotic Features**	Variable	Anhedonia, delusions (often mood-congruent), dysphoric	Antidepressant + SGAs, ECT, psychotherapy	Good with treatment, watch for recurrence
6	**Bipolar I Disorder, MRE Manic or Depressed with Psychotic Features**	Rapid, days to weeks	Irritability, grandiosity, sleep disturbance	SGAs+ mood stabilizer	Good with treatment, risk of relapse
7	**Late-Onset Schizophrenia**	Gradual, after age 40	Paranoid delusions, auditory hallucinations	SGAs[1]: 1. Risperidone 1.25–3.5 mg/d 2. Quetiapine 100–300 mg/d 3. Olanzapine 7.5–15 mg/d 4. Aripiprazole 15–30 mg/d Psychosocial support to improve functional adaptational skills[2] Cognitive behavioral therapy[2] Social skills training[2]	Often chronic, better prognosis than early-onset schizophrenia
8	**Very Late-Onset Schizophrenia-Like Psychosis**	Gradual, after age 60	Paranoid delusions, visual hallucinations	SGAs[3]: 1. Quetiapine 25–200 mg/d 2. Aripiprazole 7.5–15 mg/d Psychosocial support	Often chronic, associated with cognitive decline and very high risk of antipsychotic-induced tardive dyskinesia
9	**Delusional Disorder in Late Life**	Gradual	Delusions (persecution, jealousy, somatic)	SGAs[1]: 1. Risperidone 0.75–2.5 mg/d 2. Olanzapine 5–10 mg/d 3. Quetiapine 50–200 mg/d Cognitive therapy Psychosocial support	Chronic but less impairing than schizophrenia
10	**Schizoaffective Disorder in Late Life**	Variable	Symptoms of both schizophrenia and mood disorder (depressive or bipolar type)	SGAs + (mood stabilizer for bipolar type or antidepressant for depressed type)	Poorer than LOS and VLOSLP due to greater treatment resistance and higher rates of death from suicide

*Unless demonstrated otherwise, consider new-onset psychotic symptoms in an older adult to be due to another medical condition or substance/medication.

[1]Reinhardt MM and Cohen CL, *Curr Psychiatry Rep* 2015.

[2]Iglewicz A et al, *Psychiatr Clin N Am* 2011;34(2):295–318.

[3]Owing to the high rate of extrapyramidal symptoms in VLOSLP, lower-potency antipsychotics are recommended. The best data are for amisulpride, which is unavailable in the US (Howard R et al, *Lancet Psychiatry* 2018;5(7):553–563).

Antipsychotics in Geriatric Psychiatry

Antipsychotics are used in geriatric psychiatry to manage a number of conditions ranging from psychotic disorders to mood disorders to agitation from dementia. Their use in older adults necessitates careful consideration of their risks and benefits, given the increased susceptibility older adults have to their side effects. This fact sheet provides a guide for clinicians on the use of antipsychotics in older adults, focusing on evidence-based practices.

Table 13: **Commonly Prescribed Antipsychotics in Older Adults**

Medication	Half-Life	FDA-Approved Indications	Off-Label Indications	Common Side Effects	Starting Dose	Dose Titration	Typical Dose Range
Aripiprazole	75 hours	Bipolar disorder, major depressive disorder (adjunct), schizophrenia	Anxiety disorders, behavioral disturbances in dementia, delirium	Akathisia, insomnia, gastrointestinal issues, impulse dyscontrol	2–5 mg daily	Increase by 2–5 mg every 1–2 weeks	5–15 mg daily
Brexpiprazole	91 hours	Agitation in Alzheimer's dementia (AD), major depressive disorder (adjunct), schizophrenia		Akathisia, impulse dyscontrol, sedation, weight gain	0.5–1 mg daily	Increase by 0.5–1 mg every 1–2 weeks	2–4 mg daily; max 3 mg daily for AD agitation
Haloperidol	12–36 hours	Acute psychosis, schizophrenia, Tourette disorder	Behavioral disturbances in dementia, delirium	EPS, tardive dyskinesia, QTc prolongation	0.25–1 mg daily or BID	Increase by 0.5–1 mg every 1-3 days	1–4 mg daily
Lurasidone	18 hours	Bipolar depression, schizophrenia	Behavioral disturbances in dementia	Akathisia, nausea, sedation	20 mg daily; take with food > 350 calories	Increase by 20 mg every week; take with food > 350 calories	20–80 mg daily
Olanzapine	21–54 hours	Bipolar depression (in combination with fluoxetine), bipolar mania, schizophrenia	Behavioral disturbances in dementia, delirium	Metabolic syndrome, weight gain, sedation	2.5–5 mg daily	Increase by 2.5–5 mg every week	5–20 mg daily
Quetiapine	6–7 hours	Bipolar disorder, major depressive disorder (adjunct), schizophrenia	Anxiety disorders, behavioral disturbances in dementia, delirium, insomnia, Parkinson's disease psychosis	Orthostatic hypotension, sedation, weight gain	25 mg qHS or BID	Increase by 25–50 mg every 2-3 days	50–300 mg daily
Risperidone	20 hours	Bipolar mania, schizophrenia	Behavioral disturbances in dementia, delirium	EPS, orthostatic hypotension, hyperprolactinemia, sedation	0.25–0.5 mg daily	Increase by 0.25–0.5 mg every 2-4 days	0.5–2 mg daily

Indications for Antipsychotic Use in Older Adults

- *Behavioral and psychological symptoms of dementia (BPSD):* Agitation, aggression, psychosis (use with caution due to black box warning).
- *Bipolar disorder (BD):* For acute mania, mixed episodes, depressed episodes, and maintenance therapy.
- *Delirium:* Short-term use for severe agitation or psychosis.
- *Major depressive disorder with psychotic features:* Ordered in combination with an antidepressant.
- *Parkinson's disease psychosis (PDP):* Specific antipsychotics like pimavanserin, quetiapine, and clozapine are prescribed.
- *Schizophrenia, schizoaffective disorder, and delusional disorder:* To manage hallucinations or delusions.

Schizophrenia and Other Psychotic Disorders (In Order of Preference)

- *First-line*: Risperidone, aripiprazole, quetiapine
- *Second-line*: Olanzapine
- *Special Treatment Considerations*
  - Starting dosages for older adults should be 25% of the recommended adult dose.
  - Maintenance doses for older adults ought to be 25%–50% of the recommended adult dose.
  - Antipsychotic doses in people with early-onset schizophrenia can be reduced by 25%–50% in later life.

– Clozapine is the treatment of choice for treatment-resistant schizophrenia in younger populations but should be used cautiously in older adults due to decreased tolerability.
– Second-generation antipsychotics (SGAs) have shown efficacy in reducing symptoms and cause less extrapyramidal symptoms/tardive dyskinesia than first-generation antipsychotics.

Clinical Questions for Antipsychotic Use

Baseline assessment

- What symptoms is the patient experiencing?
- What is the patient's past psychiatric history, including previous responses to antipsychotics?
- Are there any comorbid medical conditions (eg, cardiovascular disease, diabetes, obesity) that might influence the choice of medication?
- What other medications is the patient currently taking?

Monitoring and follow-up

- How is the patient responding to the medication (symptom improvement, side effects)?
- Are there any new or worsening side effects?
- Is there any evidence of metabolic changes (weight gain, increased glucose, worsened lipid profile)?
- Is the patient experiencing any extrapyramidal symptoms (tremor, rigidity, bradykinesia)?

Table 14: **Recommended Monitoring for Antipsychotics**

Monitoring Parameter	Baseline	1 Month	2 Months	3 Months	6 Months	Annually
Body Mass Index (BMI)	X	X	X	X	X	X
Waist Circumference	X	X	X	X	X	X
HbA1c	X			X	X	X
Fasting Plasma Glucose	X			X	X	X
Fasting Lipid Panel	X			X	X	X
Extrapyramidal Symptoms (EPS)	X	X	X	X	X	X[3]
Electrocardiogram (ECG)	X[1]				X[2]	X[2]

[1] Baseline for patients with risk factors for QTc prolongation

[2] Repeat based on clinical indication (eg, if QTc-prolonging drugs are added or if the patient experiences symptoms suggestive of an arrhythmia)

[3] Thereafter administer the Abnormal Involuntary Movement Scale (AIMS) biannually

Adapted from: DeJongh BM, *Ment Health Clin* 2021;11(6):311-319.

Side Effect Management

Anticholinergic effects

- Monitor for signs of dry mouth, constipation, urinary retention, and confusion.
- Use supportive measures (hydration, laxatives) as needed.
- Consider dose reduction or switching to a different antipsychotic if severe anticholinergic effects occur.
- The SGAs with the least anticholinergic activity are aripiprazole, brexpiprazole, lurasidone, paliperidone, and risperidone.

Cardiovascular risks

- Monitor blood pressure and ECG periodically, especially in patients with pre-existing cardiovascular conditions.
- Consider dose reduction or alternative medications if significant cardiovascular side effects occur.
- Consider discontinuing the antipsychotic if QTc interval exceeds 500 ms unless cleared by cardiology.
- The antipsychotic with the least impact on QTc intervals is aripiprazole. Others with lower risk include brexpiprazole, cariprazine, and lurasidone.

Extrapyramidal symptoms (EPS)

- Regularly assess for signs of EPS, including dystonia, parkinsonism, and akathisia.
- Administer the AIMS biannually to assess for tardive dyskinesia (TD), particularly for patients on long-term antipsychotic therapy.

- Consider dose reduction or switching to a lower-potency antipsychotic such as quetiapine or clozapine if EPS/TD occurs.
- Adjunctive medications
  - Anticholinergics (eg, benztropine) help with dystonia and parkinsonism; watch for increased confusion and constipation.
  - Propranolol is effective for akathisia but watch for hypotension and bradycardia. Other, safer, options in older adults are mirtazapine (15 mg/d for ≥5 days); vitamin B6 (600–1200 mg/d for ≥5 days), and trazodone (50 mg/d for ≥5 days) (Gerolymos C et al, *JAMA Netw Open* 2024;7(3):e241527).
  - VMAT2 inhibitors are FDA-approved for TD, though limited data exists regarding their use in older adults.

Metabolic syndrome

- Metabolic syndrome increases the risk of heart disease, stroke, and type 2 diabetes. It causes an overall higher risk of death.
- Regularly monitor weight, blood glucose, and lipid profile.
- Encourage lifestyle modifications (diet, exercise).
- Consider switching to a lower-risk antipsychotic, such as aripiprazole, brexpiprazole, cariprazine, or lurasidone, if significant metabolic changes occur.
- Collaborate with primary care providers or endocrinologists for the management of diabetes, hypertension, or dyslipidemia.

Sedation

- Schedule doses to minimize impact on daytime functioning.
- Consider dose reduction or switching to a less sedating antipsychotic, if excessive sedation still occurs.
- The least sedating antipsychotics are aripiprazole, brexpiprazole, cariprazine, and paliperidone.

COMMON LATE-LIFE PSYCHIATRIC DISORDERS

Substance Use Disorders

Substance Use Disorders in Older Adults

Substance use disorders (SUDs) in older adults are a growing concern. Effective screening, assessment, and brief interventions are crucial for management. This fact sheet provides strategies for clinicians to use at the bedside or in the office, emphasizing the Screening, Brief Intervention, and Referral to Treatment (SBIRT) model (Substance Abuse and Mental Health Services Administration [SAMHSA] TIP#26, 2020).

Epidemiology

- The prevalence of SUDs in older adults is rising as baby boomers age; this generation has had shifting attitudes toward recreational drugs.
- Despite this, older adults are still more likely to suffer from alcohol and prescription medication misuse than to use illicit substances.
- Late-onset SUDs can be triggered by stressors like loneliness, chronic pain, boredom, or decreased functional ability.

Diagnosis

- DSM-5-TR criteria for alcohol and drug use disorders focus on tolerance, withdrawal, and loss of control over use (DSM-5-TR, American Psychiatric Association, 2022).
- However, DSM-5-TR criteria may not accurately identify older adults with SUDs and should be taken with a grain of salt. For example, as opposed to younger adults, older adults:
  - May not escalate their use pattern because they tend to have lowered tolerance of substances than their younger counterparts.
  - May not exhibit classic withdrawal symptoms due to masking by physiological age-related changes and cardiovascular medications. Instead, they may have lower-intensity but longer-lasting symptoms.
  - May have decreased barriers to using substances because of fewer family, work, or social obligations.
  - May not display the typical "failure to fulfill major role obligations" if they are retired or not engaged in structured activities.
  - May not realize the problems they are experiencing are from substance use, such as hypertension from alcohol use disorder.
  - May have less evident social and interpersonal issues related to substance use due to social isolation or living alone (Han BH and Moore AA, *Clin Geriatr Med* 2018;34(1):117–129).

Screening, Brief Intervention, and Referral to Treatment (SBIRT)

The SBIRT model is a comprehensive, evidence-based approach for identifying, reducing, and preventing problematic substance use. It integrates **Screening** to identify substance use behaviors, **Brief Intervention** to provide immediate counseling and motivate behavior change, and **Referral to Treatment** for individuals who require more intensive care. I will describe each of these three phases as applied to older adults.

Screening

- Use a validated tool: Choose a tool appropriate for older adults.
  - **C**ut-down, **A**nnoyed, **G**uilty, and **E**ye-opener (CAGE)
    - The CAGE questionnaire has been studied in older adults and found to have a sensitivity of 86% and a specificity of 78% (Han BH and Moore AA, *Clin Geriatr Med* 2018;34(1):117–129).
    - Two or more "yes" answers indicate a positive screen.

Table 15: **CAGE Questions**

Question	Scoring
Have you ever felt you should cut down on your drinking?	Yes/No
Have people annoyed you by criticizing your drinking?	Yes/No
Have you ever felt bad or guilty about your drinking?	Yes/No
Have you ever had a drink first thing in the morning to steady your nerves or to get rid of a hangover (eye-opener)?	Yes/No

  - **S**hort **M**ichigan **A**lcohol **S**creening **T**est-**G**eriatric Version (SMAST-G) (Blow FC et al, *Alcohol Clin Exp Res* 1992;16(2):372).
    - The SMAST-G emphasizes the older adult's relationship to alcohol and the effects of drinking. Two or more "yes" responses indicate a likely problem with alcohol (Kuerbis A et al, *Clin Geriatr Med* 2014;30(3):629–654).

Table 16: **SMAST-G Questions**

Question	Scoring
Do you ever underestimate how much you drink when talking with others?	Yes/No
After a few drinks, have you sometimes not eaten or been able to skip a meal because you didn't feel hungry?	Yes/No
Does having a few drinks help decrease your shakiness or tremors?	Yes/No
Does alcohol sometimes make it hard for you to remember parts of the day or night?	Yes/No
Do you usually take a drink to relax or calm your nerves?	Yes/No
Do you drink to take your mind off your problems?	Yes/No
Have you ever increased your drinking after experiencing a loss in your life?	Yes/No
Has a doctor or nurse ever said they were worried or concerned about your drinking?	Yes/No
Have you ever made rules to manage your drinking?	Yes/No
When you feel lonely, does having a drink help?	Yes/No

Table 17: **Comparison of Screening Tools in Older Adults**

Tool	Substances	Questions	Scoring	Use in Older Adults	Administration Time
AUDIT-C	Alcohol	3	4+ in men, 3+ in women indicates risky use	Short form of AUDIT focuses on consumption	1 minute
CAGE	Alcohol	4	2+ "yes" responses	Quick, but limited to alcohol and may miss current use or heavy and binge use	1–2 minutes
CAGE-AID	Alcohol and Drugs	4	2+ "yes" responses	Adapts CAGE for broader substance use but may miss current use or heavy and binge use	1–2 minutes
SMAST-G	Alcohol	10	2+ "yes" responses indicate likely alcohol problems	Specific for older adults, covers health and social issues	3–5 minutes

- Strategy
  - Utilize the CAGE questionnaire during initial visits or when substance use is suspected.
  - If the results of the CAGE are unclear, then administer the SMAST-G, which is more specific for older adults.
  - When using the CAGE questionnaire, keep in mind that it assesses lifetime rather than current drinking patterns. To obtain a more accurate assessment of current alcohol use, avoid asking general questions about weekly intake, as patients often underestimate. Instead, ask about drinking habits on a day-by-day basis to improve accuracy and reduce recall bias.
    - For example, ask:
      - "How much did you drink today so far?"
      - "How about yesterday?"
      - "What did you drink the day before that?"
      - "Did you drink over the weekend? How much?"
    - Clarify portions:
      - "When you say a glass, was that a small glass, a pint, or a larger pour?"
      - For beer, "Was it a bottle, can, or something larger?"
    - Sum up the total weekly intake:
      - Add up their responses and repeat it back for confirmation: "So if I add that all up, it looks like about X drinks this week. Does that sound right?"
  - Keep in mind that the National Institute on Alcohol Abuse and Alcoholism (NIAAA) recommends that older adults have no more than two drinks/day for men and one drink/day for women (https://tinyurl.com/27cx9rs2). Anything more could be indicative of problematic use.
  - A "standard drink" contains approximately 0.6 fluid ounces (or 14 grams) of pure alcohol, which is equivalent to 12 ounces of beer (5% alcohol), 8 ounces of malt liquor (7% alcohol), 5 ounces of wine (12% alcohol), or 1.5 ounces of liquor/distilled spirits (80-proof).

- Because of the brief nature of these instruments, a positive result should prompt a more thorough assessment, such as the obtaining the patient's history of substance use, tolerance, and withdrawal, as well consequences of their use and any associated social impairments.

CLINICAL PEARL: *In older adults, alcohol-related problems can present atypically, with frequent falls, memory complaints, or poor medication adherence. A thorough and structured screening process helps uncover hidden or underreported alcohol use.*

Brief intervention

- *Step 1: Establish rapport*
  - Use a nonjudgmental tone and confirm the patient's willingness to discuss their substance use.
  - SUDs are chronic medical conditions. Reduce shame by talking about substance use like any other health condition (eg, anxiety or high cholesterol).
- *Step 2: Provide feedback*
  - Share the screening results with the patient.
  - Provide psychoeducation by discussing the risks associated with continued use (eg, falls with use of alcohol or benzodiazepines, which can lead to fractures and brain hemorrhages).
- *Step 3: Enhance motivation*
  - Utilize motivational interviewing (MI) techniques to explore the patient's readiness to change.
    - This includes using open-ended questions, showing concern, avoiding arguing, and supporting the patient's belief that they can change.
    - The core principle of MI is that change is an internal process, and that people change when there is a discrepancy between their current actions and their desired results. To explore this, have patients fill out the following box:

What are my reasons for continuing use?	What are my reasons to stop using?
What do the next few years look like if I continue using?	What do the next few years look like if I stop using?

- *Step 4: Develop a plan*
  - Collaboratively develop a plan with the patient's buy-in. This might include setting goals for stopping use, scheduling follow-up appointments, or considering further treatment options.

Referral to treatment

- *Step 1: Use shared decision-making*
  - Decision-making should involve the patient in determining preferences for treatment.
- *Step 2: Identify appropriate resources*
  - Patients engaged in moderately risky behaviors can be treated with brief interventions, while patients at severe risk of harm should be referred to specialty treatment centers, including for detoxification, as appropriate.
- *Step 3: Facilitate the referral*
  - If you cannot offer treatment for an SUD, refer patients out for management, including detoxification, as needed.
  - If available, older adults respond better to age-specific SUD programming, as their experiences often differ from those of younger people.
  - SAMHSA Treatment Services Locator at https://findtreatment.gov/locator lists state-licensed substance use treatment facilities.
  - Consider also referring to mutual-help groups, like Alcoholics Anonymous (AA) or Self-Management and Recovery Training (SMART). Seniors In Sobriety (SIS) (www.seniorsinsobriety.com) is part of AA. SIS maintains an online list of senior-friendly AA meetings and provides psychoeducation (SAMHSA TIP#26, 2020).

Alcohol Use Disorder in Older Adults

Alcohol use disorders (AUDs) are increasingly prevalent in older adults. This fact sheet will discuss an evidence-based approach to management, combining medications and psychosocial treatments.

CASE VIGNETTE: *Ms. Uneke, a 72-year-old woman with a 30-year history of heavy alcohol use (four to six glasses of wine daily), experiences several falls and has a history of cirrhosis. She wants to quit drinking but struggles with cravings and anxiety when cutting down. Given the diagnosis of cirrhosis, acamprosate 333 mg three times daily is started, since it is renally cleared and does not affect liver function. Ms. Uneke is also referred for psychosocial support and counseling to aid in her recovery.*

Nonpharmacological Treatments for AUD in Older Adults

- *Cognitive behavioral therapy:* This structured approach aims to change patterns of thinking and behavior that contribute to alcohol use. It teaches coping mechanisms for managing cravings and avoiding triggers.
- *Family therapy*: This therapy involves including family members in the treatment process to improve communication, address co-dependency, and strengthen support systems.
- *Motivational interviewing*: MI is a patient-centered approach designed to increase motivation for change by exploring and resolving ambivalence. This technique helps patients identify and strengthen their own reasons for making positive changes.
- *Mindfulness-based relapse prevention (MBRP):* MBRP is a therapeutic approach that integrates mindfulness practices with cognitive behavioral strategies to prevent relapse.
- *Referral management*: This approach utilizes a clinician, such as a case manager or social worker, to assist with referrals and follow-up care. The clinician should be knowledgeable about the unique needs of older adults and familiar with age-specific community resources.
- *Support groups*: Mutual-help groups such as AA and other recovery-oriented groups offer peer support for maintaining abstinence.
- *Twelve-step facilitation (TSF)*: TSF encourages engagement with 12-step programs like Alcoholics Anonymous (AA) via promoting social support and long-term abstinence (SAMHSA TIP#26, 2020).

Table 18: **Medications to Treat AUD in Older Adults**

Medication	Titration	Initiation	Side Effects	Half-life	Dose Adjustments	Considerations in Older Adults
Acamprosate	333 mg–PO TID × 7 days, then 666 mg PO TID	When abstinence is achieved	Depression, diarrhea, flatulence	20–33 h	Adjust in renal impairment	Second-line choice, avoid in severe renal impairment or dialysis, best for older adults who cannot take naltrexone due to liver disease or concurrent opioid treatment
Disulfiram	250 mg PO daily × 1-2 weeks, then reduce to 125 mg PO daily	Abstinence from alcohol > 12 hours	Disulfiram reaction, hepatotoxicity, mania/psychosis (rare), peripheral neuropathy, rash, sedation	60–120 h	Avoid in hepatic impairment	Rarely used in older adults due to side effects, drug-drug interactions, and potential worsening of underlying medical conditions
Naltrexone IM	380 mg IM q4weeks	Free from opioids for 7–10 days	Hepatotoxicity (rare), injection-site reactions, insomnia, nausea, vomiting	5–10 days	Monitor LFTs, avoid in hepatic impairment	Unstudied in older adults; will prevent action of opioids for treatment of pain
Naltrexone PO	25 mg PO daily × 7 days, then 50 mg PO daily	Free from opioids for 7–10 days; can start while the patient is still drinking	Hepatotoxicity (rare), insomnia, nausea, vomiting	4 h	Monitor LFTs, avoid in hepatic impairment	First-line choice, only medication-assisted treatment (MAT) studied in older adults, will prevent action of opioids for treatment of pain

Medications for Alcohol Use Disorder (AUD)

Recommended treatment approach

- Oral naltrexone is the first-line choice. It is the only medication treatment studied in older adults with AUD. Avoid it in older adults taking opioid pain medications, as it will block their action, and in patients who have hepatic impairment.
- A second-line option is acamprosate, but it should be avoided in patients with severe renal impairment or in those receiving dialysis.
- Naltrexone intramuscular (IM) is a reasonable, but unstudied option, for older adults.
- Avoid initiating disulfiram in older adults due to the risk of serious adverse reactions, as well as potential medical complications, including death from a disulfiram reaction.

Naltrexone

- *Mechanism:* Opioid blocker that reduces the rewarding effects of alcohol. This results in fewer drinking days, less heavy drinking, and decreased alcohol cravings.
- *Use:* First-line treatment for AUD in older adults. It is the only MAT studied in older adults (Oslin DW et al, *Am J Geriatr Psychiatry* 1997;5(4):324–332).
- *Precautions*
  - Metabolized by the liver. Monitor liver function tests at baseline and every 6–12 months.
  - Avoid in patients with liver enzymes > 5 times the upper limit of normal or in those with underlying liver disease such as hepatitis C virus or hepatitis B core antibody.
- *Dosing*
  - Oral: 25 mg PO daily × 7 days, then 50 mg PO daily.
  - Injectable: 380 mg IM monthly.
- *Side effects:* Nausea, vomiting, insomnia, hepatotoxicity (rare), injection-site reactions with IM.
- *Considerations in older adults*
  - Interferes with opioid pain management. This can be a significant issue in medically compromised older adults who might be taking opioids for pain, arthritis, or other conditions.

Acamprosate (Campral)

- *Mechanism:* May stabilize GABA activity, thereby reducing alcohol cravings.
- *Use:* Acamprosate is best for patients who have already achieved abstinence. In younger adults, it reduces the risk of returning to drinking and increases the cumulative duration of abstinence (Witkiewitz K et al, *Ther Clin Risk Manag* 2012;8:45–53). Acamprosate can be combined with naltrexone, though this has not been studied in older adults.
- *Precautions*
  - Safe in liver disease, unlike naltrexone, but eschew it in patients with severe renal impairment.
  - Order baseline renal function tests and follow-up tests if there is evidence of impairment.
  - Acamprosate does not interact with other medications.
- *Dosing*
  - Initial: 333 mg PO TID × 7 days.
  - Maintenance: 666 mg PO TID if no side effects.
- *Side effects*: Diarrhea, flatulence.
- *Considerations in older adults*
  - Can add to pill burden (two large pills taken three times daily) for older adults who are likely already taking several other medications.
  - Best for older adults who cannot take naltrexone because of concurrent opioid usage or liver disease.

Disulfiram (Antabuse)

- *Mechanism:* Deterrent causing an aversive reaction if alcohol is consumed.
- *Use:* In highly motivated older adults who are in good health and taking few other medications. Outcomes are best if a support person can help monitor its administration.
- *Precautions*
  - Can exacerbate heart disease, diabetes, cerebrovascular disease, chronic renal failure, and peripheral neuropathy.
  - Risky in patients with cognitive impairment, poor social support, and those living alone.
  - Educate patients on avoiding all sources of alcohol and checking labels for hidden alcohol content.
- *Dosing*
  - Initial: 250 mg PO daily × one to two weeks.
  - Maintenance: 125 mg PO daily.

  (Jacobson SA, *Clinical Manual of Geriatric Psychopharmacology. 2nd ed.* Washington, DC: American Psychiatric Publishing; 2014*)*

Substance Use Disorders

- *Side effects*
  - Hepatotoxicity, mania/psychosis (rare), peripheral neuropathy, rash, sedation.
  - Disulfiram Reaction
    - Triggers
      - Consumption of alcohol: Even small amounts of alcohol found in foods, beverages, mouthwashes, aftershaves, or over-the-counter cough syrups can trigger the reaction in some individuals.
    - Symptoms
      - Mild to moderate reactions: Flushing, throbbing headache, nausea, vomiting, sweating, thirst, chest pain, palpitations, dyspnea, hyperventilation, blurred vision, and confusion.
      - Severe reactions: Hypotension, arrhythmias, myocardial infarction, acute congestive heart failure, convulsions, respiratory depression, and cardiovascular collapse.
    - Treatment
      - Immediately stop any intake of alcohol.
      - Provide supportive treatment based on the severity of symptoms.
      - Mild to moderate symptoms: Rest, hydration, antiemetics for nausea and vomiting, analgesics for headache and pain.
      - Severe symptoms: Major reactions may necessitate hospitalization. While not typically ordered by psychiatrists, treatments may include intravenous fluids, electrolytes, antihistamines, corticosteroids, and continuous monitoring of vital signs and cardiac function.
- *Considerations in older adults*
  - Disulfiram is seldom initiated in older adults with AUD because of its poor tolerability in this age group. However, I have continued it for some older adults who began taking it earlier in life and had been on it for decades.

Opioid Use Disorder in Older Adults

Opioid Use Disorders (OUDs) are increasingly prevalent in older adults. Medications for opioid use disorder (MOUD) are a critical component of OUD treatment. This fact sheet will discuss FDA-approved medications for OUD, including dosages, titration schedules, and considerations specific to this population.

Table 19: **Medications to Treat OUD in Older Adults**

Medication	Titration	Initiation	Side Effects	Half-life	Dose Adjustments	Considerations in Older Adults
Buprenorphine	Start with a test dose of 2–4 mg, increase dose in increments of 2–8 mg daily, and aim for a total daily dose of 8–16 mg	Moderate opioid withdrawal or free from opioids for several days	Confusion, constipation, hypotension, respiratory depression, sedation, sleep apnea	24–60 h	Adjust in hepatic impairment	First-line choice: It can be prescribed from an office and is less likely to interact with other medications, prolong QTc intervals, or cause respiratory depression
Methadone	Initiation and titration by a methadone clinic	Free from opioids for several days	Confusion, constipation, hypotension, QTc prolongation, respiratory depression, sedation, sleep apnea	8–59 h	Adjust in renal and hepatic impairment	Second-line choice: It may be more effective for severe OUD or in people with higher tolerance. Dispensed only from federally licensed methadone clinics. Higher risk of QTc prolongation, sedation, respiratory depression, falls, and drug-drug interactions
Naltrexone IM	380 mg IM q4weeks	Free from opioids for 7–10 days	Hepatotoxicity (rare), injection-site reactions, insomnia, nausea, vomiting	5–10 days	Monitor LFTs, avoid in severe hepatic impairment	Unstudied in older adults, will prevent action of opioids for treatment of pain
Naltrexone PO	25 mg PO daily × 7 days, then 50 mg PO daily	Free from opioids for 7–10 days	Hepatotoxicity (rare), insomnia, nausea, vomiting	4 h	Monitor LFTs, avoid in severe hepatic impairment	Third-line choice: Will prevent action of opioids for treatment of pain

Buprenorphine and Buprenorphine/Naloxone (Suboxone)

- *Forms:* Oral tablets, sublingual film, subcutaneous injection.
- *Mechanism:* Partial opioid-receptor agonist that decreases cravings and blocks full agonists like heroin.
- *Use:* First-line treatment for OUD in older adults. The recent removal of the X waiver requirement eliminates a significant prescribing barrier.
- *Considerations in older adults*
  - Can be prescribed from a clinician's office, allowing more flexibility compared to methadone. This makes it a suitable option for older adults with mobility or transportation problems since it decreases the need for frequent appointments.
  - It is less likely to interact with other medications, prolong QTc intervals, cause sedation, or trigger respiratory depression compared to full opioid agonists.
  - As with all opioids, monitor for sleep apnea, excess sedation, cognitive impairment, and falls.
  - The liver primarily metabolizes buprenorphine, and dose reductions should be considered in patients with hepatic impairment.
- *Dosing*
  - *General guidelines*
    - Buprenorphine should not be started while opioids are still in the patient's system, as this can trigger withdrawal symptoms. Instead, wait until the patient is experiencing mild to moderate withdrawal, as assessed by the Clinical Opiate Withdrawal Scale (COWS), before beginning treatment.
    - Canadian guidelines for OUD in older adults recommend reducing the initial dose by 25%–50%, lengthening dose escalation by 25%–50%, and titrating until opioid cravings are suppressed (Rieb LM et al, *CGJ* 2020;23(1):123–134).
  - *Buprenorphine and buprenorphine/naloxone*
    - The addition of naloxone prevents diversion. When Suboxone is taken as prescribed (sublingually), naloxone has minimal to no effect because it is poorly absorbed through the sublingual route. If Suboxone is dissolved and injected, naloxone becomes active and will block the action of buprenorphine, as well as precipitate opioid withdrawal.

- Initial dosing: Begin with a test dose of 2 mg buprenorphine or 2/0.5 mg buprenorphine/naloxone. If withdrawal symptoms do not worsen, an additional dose of 2–4 mg can be administered after one to two hours if symptoms persist.
  - Day 1: Aim for a maximum dose of 8 mg buprenorphine or 8/2 mg buprenorphine/naloxone.
  - Day 2 onward: Increase the total daily dose by 2–4 mg as needed until opioid cravings are suppressed.
- Maintenance dose: The target maintenance dose is typically 8–16 mg daily for buprenorphine or 8/2–16/4 mg for buprenorphine/naloxone (Crotty K et al, *J Addict Med* 2020;14(2):99–112). Some patients may require up to 24 mg daily, though this is less common in older adults.

- *Microdosing buprenorphine in older adults*
  - Rationale
    - Can help transition patients to buprenorphine from full opioid agonists like methadone, fentanyl, or heroin.
    - In this strategy, microdoses of buprenorphine are started right away and slowly increased before withdrawal begins.
    - The idea is that small doses, because of their higher receptor affinity, will gradually replace the full agonist, resulting in the patient shifting to buprenorphine without withdrawing.
    - This strategy has not been formally tested in older adults but may be a reasonable approach. It avoids florid opioid withdrawal symptoms, which can result in complications in older adults due to dehydration and kidney failure from vomiting and diarrhea.
  - Advantages
    - Reduces the risk of precipitated withdrawal.
    - Superior tolerability in older adults who have potentially lower opioid tolerance.
    - Allows for careful monitoring of side effects and therapeutic action.
  - Disadvantages
    - May be a better strategy for hospitalized older adults.
    - Mild opioid withdrawal might still occur.
    - Untested in older adults.
  - Microdosing protocol
    - Day 1: Start with 0.5 mg of buprenorphine. Continue full agonist.
    - Day 2: Increase to 0.5 mg two times a day (BID). Continue full agonist.
    - Day 3: Increase to 1 mg BID. Continue full agonist.
    - Day 4: Increase to 2 mg BID. Continue full agonist.
    - Day 5: Increase to 2 mg three times a day (TID). Continue full agonist.
    - Day 6: Increase to 4 mg BID, which is enough buprenorphine to saturate the opioid receptors fully. Stop full agonist (Personal Communication: James Sherer, MD; June 9, 2024).
    - Continue: Increase by 2–4 mg every one to two days until opioid cravings are suppressed, typically when dose is 8–16 mg daily.
- *Sublocade (buprenorphine extended-release injection)*
  - Form: Monthly subcutaneous injection.
  - Mechanism: Provides continuous release of buprenorphine over a month.
  - Use: Ideal for patients with moderate to severe OUD who have stabilized on a daily buprenorphine regimen for at least 7 days.
  - Dosing
    - Initial dose: 300 mg subcutaneously monthly for the first two months.
    - Maintenance dose: 100 mg monthly. Some patients may require a higher maintenance dose of 300 mg monthly.
  - Advantages
    - Ensures compliance with once-monthly administration.
    - Reduces the risk of diversion and misuse.
  - Disadvantages
    - Not suitable for patients who require flexible dosing adjustments.
    - Monitor older adults for sedation or respiratory depression.
    - Untested in older adults.
    - Because of the risk of serious harm or death that could result from intravenous self-administration, it is only available through SUBLOCADE REMS (Risk, Evaluation, and Mitigation Strategy). A certified healthcare professional must administer it.

Methadone

- *Form:* Oral solution or tablets.
- *Mechanism:* Full opioid-receptor agonist.
- *Use:* May be more effective for patients with severe OUD, higher tolerance to opioids, or those who could not tolerate buprenorphine or found it ineffective. It is dispensed only from federally licensed methadone clinics. This limits its use in older adults without access to transportation or who have restricted mobility.
- *Considerations in older adults*
  - Risk of QTc prolongation, sedation, respiratory depression, and falls.
  - Numerous drug-drug interactions, as it inhibits CYP2D6 and is metabolized by CYP3A4.
  - Use cautiously in patients with hepatic or renal disease.
  - The methadone clinic will manage initiation and titration.
  - Always verify the dose and that the patient is in good standing with the clinic before ordering methadone in the hospital setting.
- *Dosing*
  - Initial: 10–20 mg daily.
  - Maintenance: 60–120 mg daily.
- *Side effects:* Confusion, constipation, hypotension, QTc prolongation at higher doses, respiratory depression, sedation, sleep apnea.

Naltrexone

- *Form:* Oral or extended-release injectable (Vivitrol).
- *Mechanism:* Opioid blocker.
- *Use:* Third-line option for OUD. Consider it when opioid agonist treatment is contraindicated, unacceptable, or unavailable (Dufort A et al, *Drugs Aging* 2021;38(12):1043–1053).
- *Considerations in older adults*
  - Third-line choice behind buprenorphine and methadone.
  - Prevents action of opioids for treatment of pain.
  - Suitable for patients with sustained abstinence.
- *Dosing*
  - Oral: 25 mg PO daily × 7 days, then 50 mg PO daily.
  - Injectable: 380 mg IM monthly.
- *Side effects:* Hepatotoxicity (rare), injection-site reactions, insomnia, nausea, vomiting.

COMMON LATE-LIFE PSYCHIATRIC DISORDERS

Trauma and Stressor-Related Disorders

Post-Traumatic Stress Disorder in Older Adults

Post-traumatic stress disorder (PTSD) may develop after a person experiences or witnesses a traumatic, life-threatening event. Though nearly 90% of older adults have had trauma, only about 3% develop PTSD (Kuwert P et al, *CMAJ* 2013;185(8):685; Lee L, *PTSD Research Quarterly* 2019;30(4):1-12). PTSD can persist for decades though, often going undiagnosed in older populations, or it can present for the first time in later life.

How Aging Can Affect PTSD

- Old age can intensify PTSD symptoms due to feelings of increased vulnerability and decreased effectiveness of previous coping strategies from cognitive changes.
- Key factors include:
  - Self-reflection: Aging and retirement often lead patients to revisit the past, including traumatic memories, which can prompt PTSD.
  - Loss: The death of loved ones can remove crucial support systems, heighten feelings of loneliness and insecurity, or trigger memories of previous losses.
  - Increased screen time: Watching triggering content on TV can cause flashbacks. (https://tinyurl.com/378byfxh).
  - Medical issues: Medically induced PTSD may occur in older adults who have suffered from any of the following: cancer, multiple sclerosis, severe pain, falls, heart attacks, cardiac surgery, ICU admissions, or long-term care stays (Moye J and Rouse SJ, *Clin Geriatr Med* 2014;30(3):577-589).

Differences Between PTSD in Older and Younger Adults

- Late-life PTSD is often comorbid with depression and anxiety, though older adults are less likely to use those terms.
- Older adults may report more somatic complaints (eg, pain, GI issues, sleep difficulties) than psychological symptoms.
- Older adults who experience trauma later in life report more avoidance and sleep problems than younger adults with PTSD (Pless Kaiser A et al, *Clin Gerontol* 2019;42(4):359–376).

Table 20: **PTSD Symptoms in Older vs Younger Adults**

Symptom	Older Adults	Younger Adults
Comorbid depression	Less common	More common
Emotional numbing	Less common	More common
Hyperarousal	Less common	More common
Memory problems	More common	Less common
Somatic complaints	More common	Less common

Screening

- Ask older adults about trauma, as they may not spontaneously bring it up, especially if the trauma occurred a long time ago. They also may not connect a remote trauma with current symptoms.
- Cognitive impairment can influence a patient's ability to express symptoms. The onset of memory loss can also activate PTSD by weakening coping mechanisms.
- The PTSD Checklist for DSM-5 (PCL-5) is an effective PTSD screening scale, but it has not been studied in older adults. The checklist contains 20 self-report questions and takes 5–10 minutes to complete. It is available at: https://tinyurl.com/5n8dca9u.
- In place of administering the scale, a few screening questions are:
  - *Trauma exposure and intrusion symptoms:* "Have you ever experienced or seen a traumatic event that involved actual or threatened death, serious injury, or sexual violence?" If yes, follow up with, "Do you have nightmares about it, or do you find that you can't stop thinking about what happened?"
  - *Avoidance symptoms:* "Do you avoid thinking about or talking about the event, or do you avoid reminders of it like TV shows or news articles?"
  - *Negative alterations in cognition and mood:* "Have you changed since the event, such as believing the world is very unsafe or feeling numb to everything?"

Treatment Approaches

Psychotherapy

Trauma-focused psychotherapy is more efficacious than medications for PTSD and should be offered when possible (https://tinyurl.com/4k6jwazt).

- *Cognitive processing therapy (CPT):* Focuses on modifying distorted beliefs related to the trauma.
- *Eye movement desensitization and reprocessing (EMDR):* Comprises processing trauma-related memories while focusing on external stimuli (eg, moving fingers).
- *Narrative exposure therapy (NET):* Particularly effective for complex trauma, it involves constructing a detailed narrative of the traumatic experience.
- *Prolonged exposure (PE):* Focuses on repeated and detailed reimagining of the traumatic event in a controlled and supportive therapeutic setting. PE aims to help patients process and diminish the emotional intensity associated with the trauma by confronting distressing memories and feelings rather than avoiding them. Over time, this leads to desensitization to the traumatic stimuli, thereby reducing symptoms of distress.
- *Social support and group therapy*
  - Participation in support groups provides emotional support and reduces isolation.
  - Group therapy may be beneficial, especially when tailored to an older adult's experiences (eg, veteran's groups).

Psychopharmacology

- VA guidelines recommend sertraline, paroxetine, fluoxetine, or venlafaxine as monotherapy for older adults who choose not to engage in or are unable to access trauma-focused psychotherapy.
- Prazosin and clonidine have been used for PTSD nightmares, but in older adults, low blood pressure and falls are a concern.

Table 21: **Comparison of Medications for Treatment of PTSD in Older Adults**

Medication	Initial Dose	Dose Range	Evidence	Older Age Considerations
Sertraline	12.5–25 mg daily	12.5–100 mg daily	Moderate	• Diarrhea/nausea • Hyponatremia • Sedation • FDA-approved for PTSD
Fluoxetine	5 mg daily	5–40 mg daily	Moderate	• Hyponatremia • Long half-life • Many drug-drug interactions from CYP450 inhibition
Paroxetine	5 mg daily	5–40 mg daily	Moderate	• Anticholinergic side effects • Discontinuation syndrome • Hyponatremia • Many drug-drug interactions from CYP450 inhibition • FDA-approved for PTSD
Venlafaxine	37.5 mg daily	37.5–225 mg daily	Moderate	• Can increase hyperarousal • Discontinuation syndrome • Hypertension • Hyponatremia
Mirtazapine	7.5 mg qHS	7.5–30 mg qHS	Very Low	• Low WBCs (rare) • Sedation • Weight gain
Prazosin	1 mg qHS Monitor BP	1–6 mg qHS	Questionable	• Bradycardia • Falls • Orthostatic hypotension • Target Symptoms: Nightmares, hyperarousal
Trazodone	12.5–25 mg qHS	12.5–100 mg qHS	No Data	• Falls • Orthostatic hypotension • Target Symptom: Insomnia

Source: www.healthquality.va.gov/guidelines/MH/ptsd/; Moye J and Rouse SJ, *Clin Geriatr Med* 2014.

Grief and Bereavement in Late Life

Most older adults experience losses over their lifetime, including that of parents, siblings, partners, friends, and children. Grief refers to the emotional pain a person feels when someone the person loves is taken away. Bereavement is the process of grieving and mourning after a death.

CASE VIGNETTE: *Ms. Jones is an 82-year-old widow who lost her husband of 60 years. Six months later, she struggles to get out of bed, remains socially withdrawn, and expresses persistent guilt that she "did not do enough." Her appetite is poor, and she has lost 15 pounds. She denies suicidal ideation but reports having no desire to keep living. She has poorly controlled hypertension and often misses medical appointments because she "cannot face the world."*

Bereavement

Bereavement in older adults is associated with negative outcomes, including worsening health, weight loss, increased rates of illness, functional impairment, and increased mortality, which is highest in the first 90 days following the loss (Shear MK et al, *Curr Psychiatry Rep* 2013;15(11):406).

Grief

Prolonged grief disorder (PGD) is a condition where individuals experience persistent and intense grief affecting daily functioning, for at least 12 months after the loss. The prevalence of PGD may be as high as 1 out of 10 in bereaved older adults (Lundorff M et al, *J Affect Disord* 2017;212:138-149).

Recognizing Grief, PGD, and Depression

Typical grief

- Symptoms include sadness, yearning, guilt, anger, anxiety, nightmares, and fear.
- Grief decreases in intensity over days to months.
- People who are grieving can still experience joy.
- Grief does not impair functional ability.
- Suicidal thoughts are not present.
- Medications, eg, anxiolytics and hypnotics, may help in the short term for severe symptoms.
- Symptoms can improve on their own or with the help of therapy (Colvin C and Ceide M, *Curr Geriatr Rep* 2021;10(3):116–123).

PGD

- Intense longing or preoccupation with the deceased.
- Symptoms include emotional numbness, detachment, or bitterness regarding the loss.
- People can have intense loneliness and feel like life is meaningless as a result of the death.
- Individuals experience a lack of positive emotions.
- There is difficulty engaging in social activities or returning to usual routines.
- Symptoms persist for more than 12 months post-loss (APA, DSM-5-TR *American Psychiatric Publishing*;2022).

Major depressive disorder (MDD)

- Symptoms of MDD, grief, and prolonged grief have significant overlap.
- MDD can be diagnosed in addition to bereavement.
- In grief and PGD, distress is centered on the sense of loss and separation from a loved one, whereas in depression, it is typically linked to feelings of poor self-worth and perceived personal inadequacies.

Key questions to ask

- "Can you tell me about your loved one and what you miss the most?"
- "Have you noticed any changes in your memory, weight, or sleep patterns since your loss?"
- "Have you been feeling more anxious?"
- "What are your most troubling thoughts about your loss? Is the loss all you can think about?"
- "Are you feeling disconnected or numb?"
- "Are you still able to enjoy things?"
- "Are you able to carry on with your day-to-day activities?"
- "Do you feel supported by your friends and family during this time?"
- "Have you had any thoughts that life isn't worth living or thoughts of hurting yourself?"

Treatment for Grief and PGD

Therapy

- *Art therapy:* Uses creative processes like drawing, painting, or sculpting to help patients express their feelings and process grief.
- *Behavioral activation:* Helps individuals reengage in meaningful activities. (See "Behavioral Activation for Older Adults with Depression" [page 50] fact sheet in the "Depressive Disorders" section of this book.)
- *Complicated grief therapy (CGT):* Specialized therapy designed for PGD combining elements of cognitive behavior therapy (CBT) with grief-resolution techniques. Along with behavioral interventions, it is considered the most effective treatment for PGD in older adults (Roberts KE et al, *Curr Treat Options Psychiatry* 2019;6(4):422–449).
- *CBT*: Helpful components include grief psychoeducation, modification of dysfunctional loss-related thoughts, and development of adaptive thoughts (eg, optimistic coping with the loss and focusing on positive memories of the deceased).
- *Interpersonal psychotherapy (IPT):* Focuses on grief by addressing problems in personal relationships and poor communication patterns. Less effective for PGD than CGT in older adults (Shear MK et al, *JAMA Psychiatry* 2014). See "Interpersonal Therapy for Late-Life Depression" [page 54] fact sheet in the "Depressive Disorders" section of this book.
- *Memorializing the deceased:* Engaging in memorial activities that honor the memory of the deceased, such as planting a garden, dedicating a place in their honor, or other personalized acts, can provide a sense of legacy and continuity. Memory boxes or scrapbooks are another way for the patient to feel connected to the deceased.
- *Music therapy:* Engages patients in listening to, discussing, and creating music as a means to express emotions and facilitate healing.
- *Spiritual counseling:* Many find comfort in reconnecting with their spiritual beliefs or exploring spirituality to find meaning and solace after a loss.
- *Support groups:* Provide a space where individuals can share their experiences and feelings with others who have had similar losses. Some support groups are facilitated by professionals or peer-led, while other groups are offered through hospitals, churches, or community centers.
- *Writing or journaling:* Promotes the expression of thoughts and emotions through written words, offering a therapeutic outlet for individuals who may find it challenging to convey their feelings verbally.

When to Consider Medications

Severe symptoms

- Medications may be indicated when symptoms of PGD persist despite psychotherapy and other nonpharmacological interventions.
- Consider pharmacologic treatment if patients develop severe symptoms, such as hopelessness, feelings of worthlessness, or thoughts of suicide.
- Immediate hospitalization should be considered in cases of suicidal ideation with intent or plan.

Functional impairment

When PGD significantly disrupts daily functioning, including self-care, social relationships, or fulfilling life responsibilities, medication may help restore functionality.

Comorbid conditions

Pharmacological treatment is appropriate when PGD coexists with conditions such as MDD, severe anxiety, PTSD, severe insomnia, or other major mental health disorders. Addressing these comorbidities can alleviate suffering and support overall recovery.

Medications

Antidepressants

- *Selective serotonin reuptake inhibitors (SSRIs)*, such as sertraline and escitalopram, are commonly used due to their efficacy in treating co-occurring depression and anxiety.
- *Serotonin norepinephrine reuptake inhibitors (SNRIs),* like venlafaxine and duloxetine, are helpful when symptoms also include chronic pain or significant anxiety.
- *Bupropion* is beneficial for managing anhedonia (loss of interest or pleasure) or as an alternative for patients who cannot tolerate SSRIs.
- *Mirtazapine* is useful for patients who have low mood along with poor appetite and sleep disturbances.

When to consider short-term use of benzodiazepines or hypnotics

- *Acute insomnia:* If an older adult is experiencing severe insomnia related to acute grief, consider short-term use of hypnotics like zolpidem or eszopiclone to help them get adequate rest. Other options include trazodone, melatonin, or low-dose doxepin, which may also relieve insomnia related to anxiety or distressing thoughts of the deceased.

- *Severe anxiety:* For patients with severe anxiety or panic attacks directly related to their loss, short-term use of benzodiazepines like lorazepam or clonazepam can provide reprieve. However, these should be prescribed with caution due to the risk of dependence and other adverse effects in older adults.

Considerations

- *Apathy* can emerge in patients prescribed serotonergic antidepressants. It can complicate the grieving process by masking natural emotional responses associated with grief. Some patients may discontinue their antidepressants because they feel that the medications are not allowing them to cry or mourn properly. An alternative in these situations is bupropion.
- *Duration:* The duration for which medications are prescribed can vary. Some patients may need short-term management (a few months), whereas others might require longer-term treatment depending on their overall mental health and progress.
- *Holistic approach:* Medicines should be part of a broader, comprehensive treatment plan that includes psychotherapy and social support, as well as addresses other health issues.

Resources

- *American Association of Retired Persons (AARP)*

  Website: aarp.org/caregiving/grief-loss-end-of-life/

  Overview: Offers articles, discussions, and tools for managing grief, tailored specifically for the older adult population.

  Cost: Many articles are available at no cost.
- *GriefShare*

  Website: GriefShare.org

  Overview: A network of church-based support groups for people who are grieving the loss of someone close. The site also offers daily emails to provide comfort and resources. GriefShare has in-person and online support groups.

  Cost: $0 to $20/group
- *Therapist Aid*

  Website: therapistaid.com/therapy-worksheets/grief/none?page=1

  Overview: Contains worksheets for patients on grief psychoeducation, grief myths, the stages of grief, and the tasks of mourning.

  Cost: $0

COMMON LATE-LIFE PSYCHIATRIC DISORDERS

Other Conditions

Diagnosis and Treatment of Attention-Deficit/Hyperactivity Disorder in Older Adults

ADHD can persist into later life. It impacts approximately 3% of older adults (Michielsen M et al, *Br J Psychiatry* 2012;201(4):298–305). In this fact sheet, I will describe some of the specific challenges in diagnosing and treating ADHD in this population.

Understanding ADHD in Older Adults

- Symptoms often continue from childhood into adulthood or less commonly arise in later life.
- Older adults with ADHD exhibit more inattentiveness and have less hyperactivity-impulsivity.
- Inattention symptoms include difficulty focusing on conversations or tasks, as well as poor time management.
- Impulsivity manifests as impatience or difficulty waiting, rather than physical impulsiveness.

Diagnostic Criteria and Challenges

Diagnostic criteria

- The DSM-5-TR criteria for ADHD should be contextualized for older adults.
- For example, DSM-5-TR requires that symptoms be present before age 12, but older adults may have difficulty recalling childhood behaviors, and there may be no collateral history available to verify.
- Many older adults with ADHD were not diagnosed in childhood because the condition was less recognized decades ago.

Challenges

- There can be overlapping symptoms with other conditions such as dementia, bipolar disorder, depression, and age-related changes; see "Differentiating ADHD from Other Psychiatric Disorders in Older Adults" table.
- Age-related cognitive decline complicates the differentiation between ADHD and neurocognitive disorders.

Differentiating ADHD from dementia

- ADHD symptoms are consistent and chronic, while dementia symptoms progressively worsen.
- New onset ADHD-like symptoms in an older adult may be the first sign of neurocognitive impairment. Neuropsychological testing is advised to help differentiate between the two.

CASE VIGNETTE 1: *Mrs. Adebayo, a 70-year-old retired railroad engineer, presents with complaints of poor concentration, forgetfulness, and difficulty completing tasks. Initially suspected of having early dementia, neuropsychological testing reveals a lifelong history of inattentiveness and disorganization with intact cognition. She is diagnosed with ADHD.*

Table 22: **Differentiating ADHD from Other Psychiatric Disorders in Older Adults**

Feature	Age-Related Cognitive Decline	ADHD	Bipolar Disorder	Dementia	Depression
Onset	Gradual, associated with aging	Early childhood, often persists	Typically, adolescence or young adulthood	Late-onset, progressive	Any age, often episodic
Symptom Course	Slow, gradual decline in cognitive abilities	Chronic, fluctuating	Episodic, with manic and depressive phases	Gradual decline in multiple cognitive domains	Variable, linked to mood episodes
Inattention	Mild, impacts multitasking	Task-related, improves with structure	May occur during depressive or manic phases	Widespread, impacts daily functioning	Episodic, varies with mood
Hyperactivity	Not typical	Decreases with age, may be absent	Increased energy during manic episodes	Not typical	Not typical
Impulsivity	Not typical	Persistent, context-dependent	Impulsivity during manic episodes	Not typical	Not typical
Memory Issues	Mild, affects memory retrieval more than memory formation	Task-specific, variable	May occur during depressive and manic episodes	Progressive	Often linked to poor concentration or effort
Mood Variability	Generally stable mood	Often linked to frustration	Severe mood swings	Mood changes occur frequently	Consistent low mood
Sleep Disturbances	Occurs due to age-related changes in sleeping patterns but not predominant	Common, related to inattention	Decreased need for sleep during mania	Common, related to day-night reversal	Common, related to low mood

Source: Kooij JJ et al, *Expert Rev Neurother* 2016;16(12):1371-1381.

ADHD and Aging

Impact of aging on ADHD symptoms

- Age-related cognitive decline compounds the impairments associated with ADHD, particularly in the domains of executive function and multitasking.
- Comorbid conditions such as cardiovascular disease and diabetes can influence symptom presentation and treatment.

Functional impairment

ADHD in older adults causes significant functional impairment, impacting daily activities, social relationships, and quality of life.

CASE VIGNETTE 2: *Mr. Baker, a 68-year-old retired teacher, reports chronic disorganization and procrastination. During his retirement, he has struggled with managing household tasks and finances. He attributes this to his lifelong difficulties with attention and focus. A diagnosis of ADHD is made, and appropriate interventions are initiated.*

Treatment of ADHD in Older Adults

Pre-treatment testing

- Vital signs, especially heart rate, because stimulants can cause tachycardia.
- Check weight due to the possibility of weight loss with stimulant treatment.
- While it is not mandatory for all older adults to have an ECG (electrocardiogram) before starting a stimulant, it is recommended in patients with cardiovascular risk factors.
- Neuropsychological testing to evaluate for an underlying major neurocognitive disorder.

Pharmacological treatment

- There are no guidelines for managing ADHD in older adults, though standards for adult ADHD are in development. Here are some medication recommendations to consider.
- *Stimulants*
  - Only a few stimulants are FDA-approved for use in adults. Preferred options for older adults include:
    - Mixed amphetamine salts extended release (XR)
    - Osmotic release oral system (OROS) methylphenidate
    - Dexmethylphenidate XR
    - Lisdexamfetamine

    (Source: Dobrosavljevic M et al, *Expert Rev Neurother* 2023;23(10):883-893)
  - Some stimulants have upper age limits (eg, 55 years for lisdexamfetamine and 65 years for mixed amphetamine salts XR).
  - Amphetamines are contraindicated in people with severe cardiovascular disease. Consider a cardiovascular assessment prior to initiation in patients with a personal or family history of cardiovascular disease (Goodman DW et al, *Drugs Aging* 2016;33(1):27–36).
  - Other concerning stimulant side effects in older adults are:
    - Diminished peripheral circulation
    - Hypertension
    - Insomnia
    - Tachycardia
    - Tremor exacerbation
    - Urinary retention
    - Withdrawal fatigue
    - Worsened narrow-angle glaucoma
  - Stimulants should be avoided in patients with a history of seizures, psychosis, mania, or substance use disorders.
- *Nonstimulants*
  - Atomoxetine: FDA-approved for use in adults with ADHD. It is contraindicated in people with severe cardiovascular disease, and a cardiovascular assessment is advisable in patients with increased cardiac risk.
  - Viloxazine: FDA-approved for use in adults with ADHD.
- *Off-label treatments*
  - Bupropion: Has been used safely in older adults for other diagnoses.

- Modafinil: Little published experience.
- Guanfacine: Little published experience; can cause orthostatic hypotension and falls with injury in older adults.

- *Medication management in people with dementia*
  - *Continuation of stimulants*
    - Assess the risk-benefit ratio in patients with comorbid dementia.
    - Monitor for worsening cognitive symptoms, increased agitation/irritability, or cardiovascular issues.
- *Treatment strategy*
  - First-line: Stimulants are the most effective option.
    - Start with a low-dose long-acting agent in the mornings; titrate as needed.
    - If the patient notices that the medication is wearing off in the afternoon, either increase the morning dosage or add a low dose of a short-acting stimulant from the same drug category in the afternoon.
    - Example: A patient might be ordered Adderall XR 10 mg qAM but note difficulty focusing after 3 PM every day. In this case, add Adderall 5 mg at 2 PM daily for additional coverage.
  - Second-line: Bupropion.
  - Third-line: Atomoxetine (carries cardiovascular risks; less effective than psychostimulants).
  - Coaching, skills training, and cognitive behavior therapy may augment response to psychotropic medications.

CASE VIGNETTE 3: *Mrs. Chapman, a 75-year-old with ADHD and mild dementia, has been on methylphenidate for years. Her stimulant therapy is continued with careful monitoring, including periodic ECGs and yearly follow-ups with her cardiologist. For now, it significantly improves her focus and daily functioning, outweighing potential risks.*

Table 23: **Overview of Medications for ADHD in Older Adults**

Medication	Starting Dose	Maximum Dose	Common Side Effects	Notes
Atomoxetine	40 mg/day	80 mg/day	Cardiovascular risks, dry mouth, decreased appetite, insomnia, nausea	Nonstimulant, monitor cardiac status and hepatic function
Bupropion	150 mg/day	300 mg/day	Dry mouth, insomnia, risk of seizures, weight loss	Avoid in patients with alcohol use, eating, or seizure disorders
Dexmethylphenidate XR (Focalin XR)	5 mg once daily	20 mg/day	Appetite suppression, hypertension, increased heart rate, insomnia	Monitor for cardiovascular effects
Lisdexamfetamine (Vyvanse)	10 mg once daily	70 mg/day	Appetite suppression, cardiovascular effects, insomnia, potential for abuse	Long-acting formulation
Methylphenidate (Ritalin)	5 mg daily	20–30 mg/day in divided doses	GI issues, increased blood pressure, insomnia	Give 30–45 minutes before meals, monitor for cardiovascular issues
Mixed Amphetamine Salts XR (Adderall XR)	5 mg qAM	20–30 qAM	Cardiovascular effects, potential for abuse, insomnia	Consider cardiac screening before initiation
OROS Methylphenidate (Concerta)	18 mg once daily	54 mg/day	Appetite suppression, cardiovascular effects, insomnia	Long-acting formulation
Viloxazine	200 mg/day	400 mg/day	Cardiovascular effects, insomnia	Nonstimulant, monitor cardiovascular status

Assessment and Treatment of Neurocognitive Disorders

Assessment and Treatment of Delirium in Older Adults

Delirium is common, serious, and often underdiagnosed in older adults. It is characterized by an acute onset of confusion, fluctuation in mental status, and altered levels of consciousness. Delirium is often confused with dementia, and it is important to differentiate because the two have distinct treatments. Delirium is always due to another medical condition, which must be investigated and treated for the delirium to improve. There are three different forms of delirium:

- *Hyperactive:* Accompanied by restlessness, agitation, or refusal to cooperate with medical care. Patients may pull out IVs, be combative, or attempt to leave AMA.
- *Hypoactive:* Accompanied by reduced activity and sluggishness. In the hospital setting, clinicians are often asked to see patients with hypoactive delirium for "depression" but on assessment, it becomes clear that the main issue is confusion, not low mood.
- *Mixed level of activity:* Most common form of delirium. Individuals with mixed level of activity fluctuate between high, normal, and low levels of psychomotor activity.

CLINICAL PEARL: *Impaired attention is the most reliable indicator of delirium.*

Table 24: **Differential Diagnosis for Altered Mental Status**

Features	Delirium	Dementia	Psychosis
Core feature	Inattention	Memory loss	Break with reality
Onset	Acute	Insidious	Variable
Course	Fluctuating	Chronic, progressive decline	Chronic, with exacerbations
Duration	Hours to days	Years	Months to years
Consciousness	Altered	Normal	Normal
Attention	Impaired	Normal in early stages	Normal but may be distractible
Orientation	Fluctuating	Impaired	Normal
Hallucinations	Visual	Variable	Auditory
Medical conditions or drug toxicity	Present	Usually absent	Usually absent

Initial Evaluation

- *Clinical history:* Obtain a detailed clinical history, including the onset and duration of symptoms, pre-existing cognitive function, medication changes, and active medical conditions. Since the patient may be an unreliable historian, you may need to obtain these details from other team members and family.
- *Cognitive screening:* The hallmark of delirium is reduced ability to focus, sustain, or shift attention. This differentiates it from most other mental disorders.
  - To rapidly assess attention, ask:
    - *"Please tell me the day of the week."* The most common errors are that the patient may forget the question, provide an incorrect answer, or demonstrate delayed processing.
    - *"Please spell WORLD backward."* The most common mistake is switching the O and the R. Some patients may lose track of the task, stop prematurely, or add extra letters.
    - *"Please tell me the days of the week backwards, starting with Saturday."* The most common errors include repeating days already mentioned, skipping days, or stopping before completing the sequence, which are all signs of impaired attention and concentration.

Diagnostic Workup

While it may be tempting to "throw the kitchen sink" at the patient, it is often better to order a basic workup and add additional studies as needed.

Basic workup

- *Vital signs:* Blood pressure, heart rate, oxygen saturation, respiratory rate, orthostatic blood pressure
- *Bloodwork*
  - Complete blood count: Elevated white blood cells (WBC) could indicate an infection, though older adults will not always have a WBC response when sick.

- Basic metabolic panel (BMP): Abnormal levels of sodium and ionized calcium may contribute to confusion. Kidney dysfunction, with a BUN/cre ratio of > 20, signifies dehydration, an underappreciated cause of altered mental status (AMS) in older adults.
  - Fingerstick glucose: While glucose is part of the BMP, the results will not be available immediately. A fingerstick will reveal hypo- or hyperglycemia right away; both can cause confusion. Hypoglycemia can be quickly reversed with orange juice or crackers.
  - Liver function tests might reveal evidence of liver disease. If other signs of liver impairment are present, consider adding an ammonia level to check for hyperammonemic encephalopathy.
  - B12, folate, and vitamin D levels may show correctable nutritional deficiencies that are linked with cognitive impairment.
  - Thyroid-stimulating hormone, free T4: Both hyper- and hypothyroidism can cause altered mental status in older adults.
- *COVID-19*
- *Urine studies*
  - Urinalysis and culture can help diagnose a urinary tract infection (UTI), a common cause of delirium in older adults.
  - Urine toxicology and EtOH levels identify substance abuse. Toxicology tests, though, are prone to both false negatives and positives.
- *ECG, cardiac enzymes*: Can detect cardiac disease; ECG can establish the patient's baseline QTc interval, which, if > 500 ms, might steer you away from ordering an antipsychotic.
- *Imaging:* CT head, especially if stroke, hemorrhage, or other structural abnormalities are suspected.

Advanced workup

- *Sexually transmitted diseases (STDs)*
  - Syphilis (RPR): Order if neurosyphilis is suspected, especially in patients presenting with cranial nerve dysfunction, meningitis, psychiatric symptoms, stroke-like symptoms, or in the context of known risk factors for syphilis or an unknown sexual history.
  - HIV testing: Order in patients with risk factors for HIV, in those with signs consistent with HIV-associated neurocognitive disorders, or in those with an unexplained late-life psychiatric disorder.
- *Antinuclear antibody (ANA):* An ANA may be ordered to evaluate for autoimmune disorders, such as systemic lupus erythematosus (SLE), which can present with symptoms of delirium or psychosis. This test is typically requested when a patient has additional clinical signs suggestive of an autoimmune condition, such as joint pain, rashes, or persistent fatigue.
- *Lumbar puncture (LP):* LP can help diagnose central nervous system conditions (encephalitis, HIV, meningitis, neurosyphilis, or prion disease) all of which can cause neurocognitive disorders like delirium or dementia.
- *Electroencephalogram (EEG):* Order if seizures are suspected. EEG may also support a diagnosis of delirium by revealing generalized slowing of brain electrical activity, though this finding is nonspecific.
- *Imaging*
  - Chest X-ray if pneumonia is suspected.
  - Abdominal X-ray if constipation or other disturbances are suspected, especially in patients with dementia who cannot report accurately. Constipation will not result in delirium but may contribute to agitation.
  - Brain MRI can identify structural causes of altered mental status (eg, chronic traumatic encephalopathy, malignancy, normal pressure hydrocephalus, stroke, or subdural hematoma).

Treat the Underlying Cause

Since delirium is due to another medical condition, the most important part of management is to identify and treat the underlying cause. Environmental stressors may help trigger it or contribute to its persistence.

Environmental Interventions

Recommended for all subtypes of delirium:

- Provide frequent reorientation to time, place, and situation.
- Maintain cues for day/night (eg, opening window shades in the morning, installing wall clocks/calendars).
- Minimize nighttime interruptions (eg, vitals or blood draws).
- Place items from the patient's home environment (eg, pictures, blankets) in their room to ground them in the present.
- Maintain consistency in caregivers and staff whenever possible.
- Ensure the patient uses sensory items like hearing aids, dentures, and glasses.
- Encourage early ambulation.

- Minimize central nervous system active medications, especially anticholinergics, benzodiazepines, or opioids.

Pharmacological Treatment

- For all subtypes of delirium, though there is less evidence for this approach, attempt to regulate sleep and day-night cycles by using melatonin, ramelteon, or trazodone.
- No psychiatric medication shortens the duration of delirium or treats delirium. Utilize psychotropics only if a patient poses a risk or danger to themselves or others because of confusion or agitation. See Table 25.

Special considerations

- QTc prolongation: For patients with QTc intervals greater than 500 ms, I will order divalproex, gabapentin, or a low-dose benzodiazepine instead of an antipsychotic to manage agitation.
- Hospice care: In patients with terminal delirium, where the focus is on comfort care. The use of higher doses of haloperidol, benzodiazepines, or opioids may be appropriate.

Table 25: **Medications for Delirious Agitation**

Drug	Dose	General Information and Side Effects
Typical Antipsychotics		
Haloperidol	0.5–20 mg	• Widely used for delirious agitation or psychosis. • Use it and other antipsychotics cautiously due to potential side effects. • Available in multiple formulations: Oral solution, intramuscular injection, and intravenous injection. • Side effects include: Extrapyramidal symptoms, QTc prolongation which is greatest with the IV formulation.
Second-generation Antipsychotics		
Olanzapine	2.5–10 mg	• May work faster than haloperidol. • Available as an oral disintegrating tablet, as well as intramuscular injection.
Risperidone	0.25–2 mg	• Available as an oral disintegrating tablet, as well as oral solution.
Quetiapine	25–200 mg	• Often favored due to minimal extrapyramidal side effects. • Sedating effects can help manage sleep disturbances associated with delirium. • Preferred antipsychotic over others, including clozapine and pimavanserin, for treating delirious agitation in patients with Parkinson's disease (PD) and dementia with Lewy bodies (DLB). • Can be ordered PRN, while neither clozapine nor pimavanserin are appropriate for PRN use.
Aripiprazole	2–10 mg	• Least likely to prolong QTc intervals.
Benzodiazepines		
Lorazepam	• Start at 0.5 mg q8h PRN for patients aged 60–80 • Start at 0.25 mg q8h PRN for patients >80	• Often avoided due to the risk of worsening confusion and agitation. • May be used selectively in cases of delirium due to alcohol or benzodiazepine withdrawal; when other treatments for agitation have been ineffective; or when they are unsafe (eg, in patients with PD, DLB, or QTc prolongation).
Sedatives		
Dexmedetomidine	60–90 mcg SL or buccal initially	• Similar mechanism to clonidine, ie, alpha2-adrenergic receptor agonist. • Sometimes used in its IV form (Precedex) to prevent or shorten delirium duration in patients undergoing major surgery or receiving mechanical ventilation in the critical care setting. • New SL formulation (Igalmi) is now approved for agitation in schizophrenia and bipolar disorder. It could be used in cases of delirium in older adults, though, with careful BP monitoring.

Neurobiology of Dementia: A Brief Primer

It has likely been some time since most of us reviewed neuroanatomy. Here is a short primer on brain anatomy, highlighting how different regions contribute to cognitive and behavioral functions. This overview also explores how dysfunction in these areas leads to the symptoms commonly seen in various types of dementia.

Brain Structures

Cerebral cortex

- *Function:* The cerebral cortex is involved in higher cognitive processes such as thinking, memory, reasoning, and voluntary motor functions. It's divided into four lobes: 1) frontal, 2) parietal, 3) temporal, and 4) occipital.
- *Dysfunction in dementia:* Damage to the cerebral cortex can result in a wide range of symptoms depending on the impacted part.
  - Frontal: Dysfunction here is linked to impairment in executive function, which includes planning, organizing, sequencing, and carrying out tasks. The frontal lobe is also important for behavioral (eg, disinhibition of inappropriate conduct) and mood regulation. Executive dysfunction and personality changes are seen early in frontotemporal dementia (FTD) and later in Alzheimer's dementia (AD).
  - Parietal: Plays a vital role in spatial orientation, navigation, and object recognition. In individuals with AD, damage to this region can lead to significant challenges, such as difficulty driving without becoming lost or problems in recognizing objects or familiar environments.
  - Temporal: Crucial for memory, language comprehension, and processing auditory information. It also plays a role in recognizing faces. Damage to this area can result in memory loss, disorientation, and language difficulties.
  - Occipital: Primarily responsible for visual processing. Decline in this region can lead to impaired visual recognition, difficulty perceiving spatial relationships, or visual hallucinations, which are a hallmark feature in dementia with Lewy bodies (DLB).

Substantia nigra

- *Function:* Located in the midbrain, the substantia nigra has a vital role in the control of movement through its production of dopamine, a neurotransmitter essential for motor function, memory, mood, and pleasure.
- *Dysfunction in dementia:* Lewy bodies are abnormal deposits of alpha-synuclein protein found in the brain. In Parkinson's disease dementia (PDD) and dementia with Lewy bodies (DLB), these deposits accumulate in the substantia nigra, leading to dopaminergic neuron loss. This reduction in dopamine production results in parkinsonian symptoms, including bradykinesia, rigidity, and tremors. In DLB, Lewy bodies are also widespread in the cortex, contributing to early cognitive impairment, hallucinations, and fluctuating alertness.

Hippocampus

- *Function:* Located within the medial temporal lobe. It is crucial for the formation of new memories and for orientation to place and time. It is involved in memory consolidation, a process that takes place during sleep, whereby memories kept in short-term memory are strengthened and moved to other parts of the brain for long-term storage.
- *Dysfunction in dementia:* Hippocampal atrophy is one of the earliest structural changes in AD and is strongly correlated with short-term memory loss—specifically, the inability to encode and retain new information. This deficit is often among the first clinical signs of AD, preceding impairments in other cognitive domains.

Amygdala

- *Function:* Involved in emotional processing, including regulating fear and the fight-or-flight response.
- *Dysfunction in dementia:*
  - *AD:* Amygdalar atrophy contributes to mood swings, emotional dysregulation, and reduced affective responsiveness.
  - *DLB and PDD:* Lewy body accumulation in the amygdala can lead to heightened anxiety, panic attacks, and emotional lability.

Brain stem

- *Function:* Controls essential autonomic functions (eg, heart rate, breathing, sleep-wake cycles). It is involved in the production of neurotransmitters like serotonin, crucial for mood and anxiety regulation, and acetylcholine, important for memory and attention.
- *Dysfunction in dementia:* In DLB and PDD, Lewy bodies in the brain stem can lead to REM sleep behavior disorder (RBD) and to fluctuations in autonomic function. Acetylcholine deficits can impair attention and contribute to cognitive decline in AD and DLB.

Olfactory bulb

- *Function:* Located at the base of the brain just above the nasal cavity. It is responsible for the sense of smell and is closely linked to memory and emotion.

- *Dysfunction in dementia:* Loss of the sense of smell can be an early sign of neurodegenerative diseases like AD, PDD, and DLB. It can precede cognitive symptoms by years.

Neuroanatomy of Dementia

Alzheimer's dementia

- *Cholinergic deficits:* A significant decrease in acetylcholine, a neurotransmitter essential for learning and memory, occurs due to the degeneration of cholinergic neurons in the basal forebrain (ie, the nucleus basalis of Meynert).
- *Brain regions affected:* The hippocampus and entorhinal cortex are among the first regions affected, leading to the characteristic short-term memory loss and impairment in learning seen in people with AD.

Dementia with Lewy bodies and Parkinson's disease dementia

Brain regions affected: Abnormal deposits of alpha-synuclein, known as Lewy bodies, are found in the brains of patients with DLB and PDD. These deposits are primarily located in the cerebral cortex, substantia nigra, hippocampus, amygdala, brain stem, and olfactory bulb.

Frontotemporal dementia

- *Brain regions affected:* The frontal and temporal lobes are primarily affected, leading to symptoms such as changes in personality, behavior, and language. Unlike AD, memory is often preserved in the early stages because the hippocampus is not impacted.
- *Behavioral variant FTD (bvFTD):* Characterized by prominent behavioral changes, including apathy, disinhibition, and compulsive behaviors, due to frontal lobe atrophy.
- *Primary progressive aphasia (PPA):* Characterized by progressive language difficulties from degeneration of the temporal lobes.

Vascular dementia

Brain regions affected: The pattern of cognitive impairment in vascular dementia depends on the location and extent of the vascular lesions. Commonly impacted regions include the frontal lobes, leading to executive dysfunction, and subcortical regions, contributing to psychomotor slowing, apathy, and depression.

Clinical Implications for Patient Encounters

- *Cognitive Assessments:*
  - When evaluating a patient with suspected dementia, consider which brain regions may be affected based on their symptoms.
  - Short-term memory loss suggests hippocampal involvement, which is characteristic of AD or DLB.
  - Executive dysfunction and disinhibition may indicate frontal lobe degeneration, suggestive of FTD.
- *Behavioral Symptoms:*
  - Agitation, impulsivity, or apathy are inked to frontal lobe dysfunction (as seen in FTD or advanced AD).
  - Anxiety, panic, or emotional dysregulation suggest involvement of the amygdala and limbic system (as seen in DLB, PDD, or AD).
- Diagnostic Imaging:
  - MRI or PET scans can help differentiate types of dementia by detecting patterns of brain atrophy or hypometabolism (reduced function).
  - Hippocampal atrophy is a hallmark AD.
  - Frontal and temporal lobe atrophy or hypometabolism on PET is suggestive of FTD.
  - Occipital hypometabolism on PET is seen in DLB and may correlate with visual hallucinations.

Neurocognitive Testing for Dementia

Although the diagnosis of dementia largely depends on the patient history and interviews with the patient and their caregivers, neurocognitive testing is also essential. Some of this testing can be conducted during regular visits, but for more comprehensive and formal evaluation, referral to a neuropsychologist may be necessary.

Quick Screening Tests for Dementia

You or your staff can administer a quick cognitive screening test in the office with your patients. It is helpful to become familiar with some of these and then choose the one that fits your style and practice. My preferred test is the Montreal Cognitive Assessment (MoCA), though the Mini-Mental State Examination (MMSE) is more helpful for staging dementia as mild, moderate, or severe.

MMSE

- *Purpose:* Assesses general cognitive impairment.
- *Administration*
  - Orientation: Ask for the date and the location.
  - Registration: Name three objects and ask the patient to repeat them.
  - Attention and calculation: Ask the patient to count backward from 100 by sevens or spell WORLD backward.
  - Language: Ask the patient to name objects, repeat phrases, and follow a three-step command.
  - Recall: Ask for the three objects named earlier (Folstein MF et al, *J Psychiatr Res* 1975;12(3):189-198).
- *Scoring:* Out of 30. Scores ≤24 suggest cognitive impairment; 18–24: mild impairment; 12–17: moderate impairment; < 12: severe impairment.
- *Usefulness:* Widely used, quick to administer (~10 minutes).
- *Limitations*
  - Less sensitive in detecting mild cognitive impairment (MCI) and early dementia.
  - Less accurate at the extremes of education.
  - Does not test executive function and is less sensitive for dementias impacting higher-order thinking, such as frontotemporal dementia (FTD).
  - Copyrighted, and in some cases, the copyright is being enforced.

MoCA

- *Purpose:* Detects MCI and mild dementia.
- *Administration*
  - Visuospatial/executive function: Draw a clock, copy a cube, connect letters and numbers sequentially.
  - Naming: Identify animals.
  - Short-term memory: Repeat a list of words and recall them later.
  - Working memory/attention: Repeat a series of numbers backward.
  - Attention: Tap hand at a specific letter in a list of letters.
  - Language: Repeat sentences and name animals starting with a given letter.
  - Abstraction: Explain the similarity between two objects.
  - Orientation: Ask the date and location.
- *Scoring:* Out of 30. Scores <26 suggest cognitive impairment.
- *Usefulness:* MoCA is more sensitive than the MMSE in detecting MCI, with a sensitivity of 90% compared to 60% for the MMSE (Nasreddine ZS et al, *J Am Geriatr Soc* 2005;53(4):695-699).
- *Limitations*
  - Takes longer than the MMSE (~10-15 minutes).
  - Copyrighted, a one-hour online training and certification module is required.

Saint Louis University Mental Status exam (SLUMS)

- *Purpose:* Screens for MCI and dementia.
- *Administration*
  - Orientation: Ask about the date and location.
  - Calculation: Subtraction and addition tested.
  - Language/verbal fluency: Name as many animals as possible in one minute.
  - Short-term memory: Recall five words.
  - Working memory/attention: Repeat a series of numbers backward.
  - Executive/visuospatial function, short-term memory: Draw a clock with hands pointing to 10 minutes to 11.

- Executive/visuospatial function: Identify a triangle and place an X in the largest of three figures.
- Immediate recall/memory, executive function: Answer questions about a short vignette

- *Scoring:* Out of 30. Scores <27 suggest MCI, <21 indicates dementia.
- *Usefulness*
  - More comprehensive than other short scales.
  - Detects MCI better than the MMSE (Tariq SH et al, *Am J Geriatr Psych* 2006;14:900-910).
  - Free to use.
- How to access: The test and an instructional video can be found at https://tinyurl.com/4vavx6n8.

Neuropsychological Testing

Why and when to order

- Neuropsychological testing is the gold standard for diagnosing dementia. Some clinicians are skeptical of its utility because it is onerous to patients and often not readily available. After all, if you have done a careful evaluation of the patient and family as suggested, and all signs point to dementia, what is the point of insisting on more testing? In my experience, the testing is particularly helpful for the following reasons.
- *Diagnosis*
  - DSM-5-TR requires that cognitive impairment be exhibited in one or more domains to diagnose mild or major neurocognitive disorder that is "preferably demonstrated by neuropsychological assessment or other quantifiable means" (APA, DSM-5-TR *American Psychiatric Publishing*;2022).
  - It can help if you are uncertain about the diagnosis.
  - It discriminates between different types of dementias (ie, it differentiates between normal aging, MCI, and dementia), or determines if other psychiatric disorders, such as depression or psychosis, are impacting the presentation.
- *Baseline measurement:* It provides an objective baseline measurement before starting treatment, allowing you to monitor cognition over time. This is also useful in cases of MCI, as many patients will progress to dementia.
- *Legal and occupational reasons:* Neuropsychological testing's relative objectivity can help inform difficult issues such as competency to make medical or financial decisions or fitness for work.

How to decipher the neuropsychological testing report

- Testing reports are usually long and technical and can be difficult for clinicians to absorb and understand quickly. Scores are often presented as standard scores, percentiles, or z-scores. Results significantly below the average range suggest potential cognitive deficits in that area. The following primer will help explain some common testing domains.
- *Complex attention*
  - The capacity to maintain and manage attention over prolonged periods, particularly when handling multiple tasks simultaneously.
  - Characteristics
    - Difficulty sustaining focus on tasks.
    - Trouble shifting attention between tasks.
    - Easily distracted by irrelevant stimuli.
  - Example: A patient may find it hard to follow conversations in noisy environments or get distracted while driving, causing them to lose focus on the traffic in front of them.
- *Early behavioral changes*
  - Alterations in behavior and personality that occur early on in certain types of dementia that impact the frontal lobes.
  - Characteristics
    - Increased irritability, apathy, or social withdrawal.
    - Changes in mood, such as depression or anxiety.
    - Engaging in socially inappropriate or impulsive behaviors.
  - Example: A patient previously known for being outgoing and sociable becomes withdrawn and disinterested in social activities.
- *Executive dysfunction*
  - A disruption in managing and regulating cognitive processes that facilitate goal-directed behavior.
  - Characteristics
    - Poor planning and organizational skills.
    - Difficulty with problem-solving and decision-making.

- Example: A patient may have trouble organizing daily activities, managing finances, or following complex instructions.

- *Language impairment*
  - Difficulty with verbal and written communication, affecting the ability to understand language, speak fluently, or repeat words and phrases.
  - Characteristics
    - Problems finding the right words or naming objects (anomia).
    - Difficulty understanding spoken or written language.
    - Challenges in constructing sentences or maintaining a coherent conversation.
  - Example: A patient might struggle to follow conversations, frequently pause to find words, or produce sentences that do not make sense.
- *Short-term memory loss*
  - A deficit in the ability to hold and manipulate information for short periods, typically seconds to minutes.
  - Characteristics
    - Difficulty remembering recent events or conversations.
    - Frequently repeating questions or statements.
    - Misplacing items and being unable to retrace steps.
  - Example: A patient may forget what they ate for breakfast or the details of a recent conversation.
- *Visuospatial difficulties*
  - Impairment in the ability to appreciate visual and spatial relationships.
  - Characteristics
    - Problems with depth perception and judging distances.
    - Challenges with tasks such as navigating or assembling objects.
  - Example: A patient may struggle to find their way around their home, have trouble parking their car, or get lost driving in familiar areas.

Table 26: **Neuropsychological Domains Affected in Dementia Types**

Dementia Type	Key Cognitive Domains Affected
Alzheimer's Dementia	Short-term memory, visuospatial function, language
Frontotemporal Dementia	Personality and behavior, executive function, language
Lewy Body Dementia	Visuospatial function, executive function, attention, fluctuating cognition, less severe memory deficits than Alzheimer's dementia
Mixed Dementia	Combination of Alzheimer's and vascular features
Parkinson's Disease Dementia	Executive function, visuospatial abilities
Vascular Dementia	Executive function, complex attention, processing speed

Alzheimer's Dementia: Diagnosis and Evaluation

Alzheimer's Dementia (AD) is the most common type of dementia, comprising about 60%–70% of all dementia cases and impacting 6.2 million Americans over age 65.

Diagnostic Criteria

The following criteria are adapted from the National Institute on Aging and the Alzheimer's Association. Unlike DSM-5-TR, these criteria do not require memory loss as a symptom, allowing for the diagnosis of other AD subtypes.

- *Significant cognitive decline* reported by the patient, an informant, or observed by the clinician and documented by formal or informal neuropsychological testing.
- *Impaired independence* in daily activities.
- *Deficits in two or more of the following cognitive areas:*
  - Memory**,** especially the ability to remember new information. This is characterized by repetitive questions, losing belongings, or forgetting important events or appointments.
  - Reasoning and managing complex tasks that require executive function (ie, the ability to plan, organize, and sequence activities).
  - Visuospatial abilities, such as difficulty recognizing faces or places. People may have problems with previously known skills (eg, using tools and implements like knives and forks). There may be increased difficulty driving in familiar environments without getting lost or making errors. Patients might become more confused in the evenings and at night, called "sundowning."
  - Language function, causing difficulty speaking, reading, writing, naming objects (anomia), and repeating phrases.
  - Personality, behavior, or comportment, such as decreased motivation, apathy, social withdrawal, loss of empathy, compulsive behaviors, and socially unacceptable behaviors (eg, cursing or inappropriate sexual behavior/ comments).
- *Insidious onset and a gradual, progressive decline*
- *No evidence of another medical condition* that could substantially contribute to the presentation (McKhann GM et al, *Alzheimer's Dement* 2011;7(3):263-9).

Risk Factors

- *Age:* Most significant risk factor.
- *Sex*: Women are more likely to develop AD than men.
- *Genetics*
  - Familial Alzheimer's disease (FAD) accounts for less than 1% of cases and is associated with mutations in APP, PSEN1, or PSEN2 genes. It has autosomal dominance inheritance.
  - Patients with FAD develop AD before the age of 65 and often have a family history of early-onset AD.
  - Genetic testing is used to diagnose FAD. Given that a positive result will impact not only the patient but also their family and future generations, involving a genetic counselor is recommended.
  - Apolipoprotein E (APOE) ε4 allele increases AD risk and lowers the age of onset. It is not routinely ordered unless the patient is considering an anti-amyloid therapy.
- *Health:* Hypertension, diabetes, hypercholesterolemia, hearing loss, history of head injuries, and depression.
- *Lifestyle factors:* Smoking, physical inactivity, and poor diet.
- *Education:* Lower educational attainment.

Pathophysiology

- *Amyloid plaques:* Formed of extracellular deposits of amyloid beta peptide; Aβ40 (amyloid beta peptide 40, consisting of 40 amino acids) is expressed in healthy neurons, while Aβ42 (consists of 42 amino acids) is prone to forming plaques. Aβ42 is the key pathologic form of amyloid-beta involved in AD. Amyloid beta plaques cause neuronal cell death and disrupt neural pathways.
- *Neurofibrillary tangles*: Intracellular aggregates of hyperphosphorylated tau protein (p-tau). Buildup of p-tau correlates with functional and cognitive decline. Specific forms of pathologic p-tau can be tested in cerebrospinal fluid (CSF) and plasma. High plasma levels of p-tau181, p-tau217, and p-tau231 have been correlated with autopsy-confirmed cases of AD (Dark HE et al, *Arch Clin Neuropsychol* 2024;39(3):313-324).

Recommended Clinical Approach to Diagnosing AD

History

- Diagnosis is primarily clinical and rests on detailed patient history, focusing on changes in cognition and functioning over time.
- It is essential to establish that these are cognitive changes from baseline. For instance, a patient may not do the finances because their partner has always done them. This would not be considered a change.

Collateral history

- Since the patient is presenting with a potential cognitive disorder, they may be an inaccurate historian. Gathering collateral history from someone who knows the patient is critical.
- Most geriatricians will insist that a family member accompany the patient to a memory disorder evaluation.
- It is typical to interview the patient and the collateral informant together but consider talking to them separately if the patient is suspicious of the caregiver or very defensive.

Diagnostic tools

- Evaluation should always be accompanied by diagnostic testing. In most cases, this is to rule out another cause for the memory complaint. A brain MRI or head CT are necessary components of the evaluation.
- Neuropsychological testing is the gold standard for diagnosing dementia. If not available, complete an in-office cognitive evaluation. Most take about five to seven minutes. Recommended tools are the Montreal Cognitive Assessment (MoCA), the Saint Louis University Mental Status exam (SLUMS), or the Mini-Mental State Examination (MMSE). My preferred test is the MoCA.

Biomarkers

- Biomarkers can support a diagnosis of AD, but for now, their use is limited. PET imaging is expensive and lumbar punctures are invasive. Confirmatory tests are mainly ordered to determine eligibility for Aβ-specific therapies or if the diagnosis is unclear.
- AD biomarkers
  - Amyloid PET
  - CSF Aβ 42/40
  - CSF p-tau 181/Aβ 42
  - CSF t-tau/Aβ 42
- Blood-based biomarkers for AD have advanced considerably. A plasma p-tau217 assay has demonstrated diagnostic accuracy comparable to amyloid PET imaging and CSF biomarkers (https://tinyurl.com/2b857xvr). The FDA has authorized the pTau217/β-amyloid 1-42 plasma ratio for early detection of amyloid plaques associated with AD. In clinical validation studies, 92% of individuals with positive results had confirmed amyloid plaques on PET imaging or CSF testing, while 97% of those with negative plasma results had no evidence of amyloid on PET or CSF tests (https://www.fda.gov/news-events/press-announcements/fda-clears-first-blood-test-used-diagnosing-alzheimers-disease, Accessed May 17, 2025). The FDA has approved pTau217/ß-Amyloid 1-42 Plasma Ratio for the early detection of amyloid plaques associated with AD. In a clinical study, 92% of individuals with pTau217/ß-Amyloid 1-42 Plasma Ratio positive results had the presence of amyloid plaques by PET scan or CSF test result, and 97.% of individuals with negative results had a negative amyloid PET scan or CSF test result.

AD Variants

There are three less common forms of AD. While their presentations differ from classic AD, their underlying pathophysiology is still characterized by amyloid beta plaques and tau pathology.

1. *Frontal variant of AD*
   - Frontal variant of Alzheimer's disease (fvAD) is portrayed by apathy, disinhibition, executive dysfunction, impatience, impulsivity, irritability, and loss of empathy.
   - Although both behavioral variant frontotemporal dementia (bvFTD) and fvAD can manifest similar behavioral disturbances, bvFTD most often arises in individuals younger than 65 and patients do not have the pronounced memory deficits characteristic of fvAD.
   - Neuroimaging and biomarker studies can also aid in distinguishing between the two disorders.
2. *Posterior cortical atrophy (PCA)*
   - *Visuospatial dysfunction:* Difficulty understanding where objects are in space.
   - *Balint syndrome:* Trouble with eye movements, reaching for objects, and seeing more than one object at a time.
   - *Gerstmann syndrome:* Problems with writing, math, finger recognition, and distinguishing left from right.
   - *Visual agnosia:* Difficulty recognizing objects by sight.
   - *Apraxia:* Trouble with coordinated movements despite intact muscle strength (eg, problems buttoning a shirt correctly despite having the strength to do it).
   - *Preserved memory and insight.*
3. *Logopenic variant primary progressive aphasia (lvPPA) due to AD*
   - Often associated with AD and primarily affects language abilities.
   - Patients experience early problems with language, particularly logopenic aphasia, characterized by difficulty finding words (anomia) and impaired ability to repeat phrases.
   - Grammar and sentence structure (syntax) remain intact.
   - To distinguish lvPPA from the language impairments seen in people with FTD, particularly its primary progressive aphasia (PPA) variant, clinicians should look for preserved grammar and syntax in people with lvPPA. In contrast, patients with FTD PPA have more profound language and behavioral deficits.

When to Refer to a Neurologist?

Complex or atypical presentations

- When the patient exhibits atypical symptoms, such as rapid progression, motor changes, young onset, or if there is uncertainty about the diagnosis.
- Rapid progression: AD progresses over years. Rapid progression is considered significant deterioration of memory and functioning within 6–12 months and might be due to another etiology.

Need for advanced diagnostic testing

In most cases, this will be for CSF testing or electroencephalography (EEG) to rule out a seizure disorder or encephalopathy. PET, SPECT, genetic tests, and blood biomarkers can all be ordered by psychiatrists.

When to Tell Patients and Families?

- As soon as you are ready to make a diagnosis, you should disclose it to the patient and their family, so they can begin processing and planning.
- In many cases, the diagnosis will not be a surprise; after all, the patient came for a memory evaluation, but it can still be upsetting once the diagnosis is "official." It is important to be sensitive in these conversations and allow time for the patient and family to grieve. This could also be an opportunity to refer them to the Alzheimer's Association and support groups.
- Consider spending extra time answering questions and schedule a sooner follow-up.

Alzheimer's Dementia: Stages and Treatment

Alzheimer's Dementia (AD) is a progressive neurodegenerative disorder that primarily impacts older adults. AD is characterized by three stages (mild, moderate, and severe), each with its own features and treatment strategies.

Table 27: **Stages of Alzheimer's Dementia**

Stage	Findings		Treatment
Early stage (Mild) (2–4 years)	Impaired short-term memory, not obvious to casual observers	Good memory for events in the distant past	1. Lifestyle Changes a. Cognitive and physical exercise b. Consult eldercare attorney c. Social activity d. MIND* diet 2. Nonpharmacological Treatment a. Caregiver education b. Music therapy c. Validation therapy 3. Medication Therapy a. Acetylcholinesterase inhibitor b. Anti-amyloid monoclonal antibody
	Mild disorientation to time and place and word-finding difficulties	Some losses in instrumental ADLs, (eg, driving, meal preparation, finances)	
	Subtle social withdrawal or passivity	Self-care is preserved	
	Few behavioral manifestations	Social graces are retained	
Middle stage (Moderate) (2–10 years)	Obvious short-term memory impairment	Greater language impairment with word-finding and naming difficulty	1. Lifestyle Changes a. Cognitive and physical exercise b. Consult eldercare attorney c. Driving assessment d. MIND* diet e. Social activity 2. Nonpharmacological Treatment a. Caregiver education b. Music therapy c. Simulated presence therapy d. Validation therapy 3. Medication Therapy a. Acetylcholinesterase inhibitor b. NMDA receptor antagonist
	Apraxia manifests (difficulty buttoning shirts or brushing teeth)	Obvious impairment in instrumental ADLs (eg, paying bills or driving)	
	Visuospatial deficits (may become lost or wander)	Difficulty in self-care (eg, resistance to bathing)	
	Behavioral complications (sundowning, depression, apathy)	Variable social skills, more passive in social interactions	
Late stage (Severe) (1-3 years)	Memory in fragments only, impaired short-term and long-term memory	Diminished language output	1. Lifestyle Changes a. Cognitive exercise b. MIND diet c. Social activity 2. Nonpharmacological Treatment a. Caregiver education b. Music therapy c. Simulated presence therapy 3. Medication Therapy a. Acetylcholinesterase inhibitor b. NMDA receptor antagonist
	Significant disorientation to time and place	Need help with basic self-care—toileting, dressing, or showering; reduced mobility and incontinence	
	Disturbed sleep-wake patterns	Agnosia (trouble recognizing familiar people)	
	Significant behavioral changes such as marked apathy or hostility; delusions emerge in 20%–40%	Loss of social graces	

*Mediterranean-DASH Intervention for Neurodegenerative Delay Diet (MIND Diet)

CASE VIGNETTE 1: Early stage—*Mrs. Walker, a 72-year-old retired teacher, is having trouble remembering recent conversations and appointments. Her family notices she frequently misplaces items and struggles with planning her grocery shopping. On the Montreal Cognitive Assessment (MoCA) scale, she scores 23/30, indicating mild impairment. MRI shows mild atrophy in the medial temporal lobes. She is diagnosed with early-stage AD and started on donepezil 5 mg qAM, alongside daily memory exercises.*

CASE VIGNETTE 2: Middle stage—*Mr. Lee, an 80-year-old former engineer, presents with significant memory loss, confusion, and difficulty recognizing friends and family. His wife reports he has started wandering and has become lost while walking alone in their neighborhood. His Mini Mental State Examination (MMSE) score is 16/30, and his MRI reveals hippocampal atrophy. He begins taking donepezil and later is started on memantine. His wife is referred to a support group for caregivers.*

CASE VIGNETTE 3: Late stage—*Ms. Shah, an 85-year-old woman, is brought to the clinic by her daughter in a wheelchair. Ms. Shah can no longer recognize her daughter or other family members. She does not answer any questions posed to her. She requires assistance with all daily activities. Her Mini-Mental Status Exam score is 5/30. The focus of her care shifts to palliative measures, ensuring comfort and dignity in the final stage of AD.*

Neuropsychiatric Symptoms (NPS)

- Over 85% of older adults with dementia will develop NPS at some point and about 50% of patients will have at least four neuropsychiatric symptoms simultaneously. NPS are an expected part of the disease.
- The most common NPS, in order of frequency, are:*
  - Apathy/indifference [page 136]
  - Depression [page 138]
  - Agitation [page 129] and [page 130]
  - Irritability
  - Delusions [page 139]
  - Anxiety
  - Hallucinations [page 139]
  - Euphoria

  *See other fact sheets in this section ("Assessment and Treatment of Neurocognitive Disorders") for more on these NPS.
- Aggression and agitation can include verbal agitation—yelling, screaming, cursing; non-verbal agitation—pacing, wandering, sundowning; or physical aggression—hitting, slapping, punching, grabbing or pushing caregivers, throwing objects, biting, kicking, or scratching.
- The prevalence and severity of NPS increase as dementia progresses, often correlating with cognitive decline.

Lifestyle and Nonpharmacological Interventions

- *Caregiver education:* Provide information and support to caregivers about the disease and management strategies.
- *Cognitive stimulation:* Engage patients in activities designed to improve cognitive function, such as Sudoku, word searches, and crossword puzzles.
- *Diet:* Recommend the MIND diet, which is rich in fruits, leafy vegetables, whole grains, lean meats, and healthy fats.
- *Driving assessment:* Evaluate the ability of the individual to continue driving safely.
- *Elder care attorney:* Suggest that the patient meet with an eldercare attorney to address long-term care planning, decision-making, and healthcare directives.
- *Music therapy:* Use music to improve mood and cognitive function. Patients often respond best to music from their youth.
- *Physical exercise:* Have patients engage in regular aerobic, strength, and balance training.
- *Simulated presence therapy:* Use recordings or videos of loved ones to reduce anxiety and agitation.
- *Sleep hygiene:* Address sleep disturbances and promote good sleep habits.
- *Social activity:* Encourage participation in social and community activities.
- *Validation therapy:* Teach caregivers to communicate with empathy to validate the emotions and experiences of the person with AD, rather than contradict or argue with them.

Pharmacological Treatments FDA-Approved for AD

Anti-amyloid monoclonal antibodies (mAbs)

- *Utility:* mAbs are not recommended as first-line therapy for AD due to safety concerns (eg, brain edema and hemorrhages) and limited efficacy. However, they may be considered for carefully selected patients with amnestic mild cognitive impairment (aMCI) or early-stage AD who are highly motivated to receive a disease-modifying therapy.
- *Lecanemab (Leqembi)*
  - Mechanism: Monoclonal antibody targeting amyloid beta protofibrils.
  - Indications: Mild cognitive impairment (MCI) and mild dementia due to AD with confirmed Aβ pathology via diagnostic testing.
  - Side effects: Infusion-related reactions, headache, amyloid-related imaging abnormalities (ARIA) including 30% risk of cerebral edema and hemorrhages.
  - Efficacy: Slows, but does not stop or reverse, cognitive and functional decline. This slowing equates to 4–5 months of delay in disease-related clinical progression over 1.5 years (Ramanan VK et al, *Neurology* 2023;101(19):842-852).
  - Considerations
    - The long-term impact of ARIA is unknown.
    - Do not use in people who are Apoε4 homozygotes or taking anticoagulants because of a much higher risk of ARIA.

- Administered by infusion q2weeks.

- *Donanemab (Kisunla)*
  - Mechanism: Monoclonal antibody targeting a modified form of amyloid beta.
  - Indications: MCI due to AD and mild AD with confirmed Aβ pathology via diagnostic testing.
  - Side effects: ARIA, headache, infusion reactions.
  - Efficacy: Slows, but does not stop or reverse, cognitive and functional decline.
  - Considerations
    - The long-term impact of ARIA is unknown.
    - Do not use in people who are Apoε4 homozygotes, taking anticoagulants, or have high p-tau burden.
    - Administered by infusion q4weeks.

Cholinesterase inhibitors: Donepezil, rivastigmine, galantamine

- *Mechanism*: Increases acetylcholine levels, which helps with attention and memory.
- *Indications*: Mild, moderate, severe AD.
- *Side effects:* Nausea, vomiting, diarrhea, bradycardia, weight loss, falls.

NMDA receptor antagonist: Memantine

- *Mechanism*: Modulates glutamate activity to prevent neuronal cell death.
- *Indications*: Moderate and severe AD.
- *Side effects:* Dizziness, headache, constipation.

Recommended Approach to Pharmacologic Treatment of AD

Mild AD

- *First-line* (acetylcholinesterase inhibitor)
  - Donepezil 5–10 mg daily; a 23 mg dose is available, though it is associated with limited additional benefit and substantially more side effects.
  - Rivastigmine 3–6 mg BID or 4.6-9.5 mg TD daily.
  - Galantamine ER 16-24 mg qAM.
- *Second-Line* (anti-amyloid monoclonal antibody)
  - Donanemab or lecanemab in highly motivated patients who are not on anticoagulant treatment, have lower p-tau levels, are not Apoε4 homozygotes, and have milder symptoms.

Moderate AD

- *First-line* (acetylcholinesterase inhibitor): Acetylcholinesterase inhibitors provide more benefit than memantine in slowing disease progression.
- *Second-line* (NMDA receptor antagonist)
  - Memantine titrated to 10 mg BID or to XR 28 mg daily.
  - Combine an acetylcholinesterase inhibitor with memantine for maximum benefit.

Severe AD

- *First-line* (acetylcholinesterase inhibitor)
- *Second-line* (NMDA receptor antagonist): Combine an acetylcholinesterase inhibitor with memantine for maximum benefit.
- *In patients with severe dementia* who can no longer perform basic activities of daily living and are unable to communicate, the continued use of cognitive enhancers may not provide meaningful benefit and should be reassessed.

Dementia with Lewy Bodies: Diagnosis

Lewy Body Dementia (LBD) is a progressive neurodegenerative disorder. It is the third most common type of dementia after Alzheimer's dementia (AD) and vascular dementia. It affects approximately 1.4 million people in the US (Kane JPM et al, *Alzheimer's Res Ther* 2018;10:19). LBD includes two related conditions: 1) dementia with Lewy bodies (DLB) and 2) Parkinson's disease dementia (PDD). Both are characterized by Lewy bodies but have different presentations.

Pathophysiology

Patients with LDB have abnormal deposits of alpha-synuclein protein in the brain. These are known as Lewy bodies. In DLB, Lewy bodies are distributed throughout the brain, while in PDD they start in the substantia nigra, where they first impact movement.

Clinical Presentation of Dementia with Lewy Bodies

Core clinical features

- *Fluctuating cognition:* Marked variations in attention and alertness.
  - Questions for patients
    - "Do you have times of the day when you feel more alert or more confused?"
    - "Have you had any episodes where you suddenly become very confused or sleepy?"
  - Questions for caregivers
    - "Have you noticed random staring episodes or blank expressions?"
    - "Does the patient have periods where they seem very confused or stop making sense, followed by other times when they're more lucid?"
- *Visual hallucinations:* Detailed and recurrent visual hallucinations.
  - Many patients with DLB have awareness of their hallucinations and are not disturbed by them.
  - Questions for Patients
    - "Do you see things that aren't really there, such as people, animals, or objects?"
    - "Are they disturbing or frightening?"

CASE VIGNETTE 1: *Mr. Edelman, a 76-year-old former engineer, describes seeing small animals scurrying around his living room several times a week. These hallucinations are vivid and detailed, often causing him to trip or bump into furniture as he tries to avoid them. His wife confirms that he seems to interact with these nonexistent creatures, which has been distressing for both of them. He has also had memory issues and recently forgot his daughter's birthday.*

- *REM sleep behavior disorder (RBD):* Acting out dreams, often violent.
  - When we dream, all our muscles are paralyzed, except for our breathing muscles. This serves as a protective mechanism to keep us from acting out our dreams. However, in RBD, this paralysis is lost, allowing people to physically enact their dream content.
  - Questions for patients
    - "Do you act out your dreams, including talking, yelling, or moving around?"
    - "Have you been told that you seem to be fighting or running in your sleep?"
  - Questions for caregivers/partners
    - "Have you observed them acting out their dreams while sleeping?"
    - "Do they have violent movements or seem to be fighting in their sleep?"
    - "Have you been hurt? Do you sleep in separate beds?"

CASE VIGNETTE 2: *Mrs. Freeman, a 72-year-old retired accountant, has been acting out her dreams for the past year. Her husband reports that she has punched and kicked him in her sleep. When asked, Mrs. Freeman recalls vivid dreams in which she is fighting off robbers. A sleep study confirms the presence of RBD, and her symptoms otherwise align with a diagnosis of DLB.*

- *Parkinsonism:* Any one of either bradykinesia, rigidity, tremor, or gait abnormality.
  - Questions for patients
    - "Have you experienced any slowness of movement, muscle stiffness, or difficulty with balance?"

    - "Do you have any tremors, especially when your hands are at rest?"
  - Questions for caregivers
    - "Have you noticed any changes in their walking, such as shuffling or difficulty starting to move?"
    - "Do they seem to have muscle stiffness or slowness in their movements?"
  - Exam
    - *Bradykinesia (slowness of movement)*: Ask the patient to perform rapid alternating movements (eg, tapping the thumb and each finger together quickly; opening and closing the hands). Look for slowness in initiating, maintaining, and performing these movements.
    - *Facial expression (hypomimia)*: Look for reduced facial expressiveness, often described as a "masked" face.
    - *Gait abnormalities:* Observe the patient walking across the room, turning, and returning. Look for a shuffling gait, reduced arm swing, and difficulty rotating, such as taking multiple small steps to turn, ie, en bloc turning.
    - *Micrographia:* Ask the patient to write a sentence, which is also one of the tests on the Mini-Mental State Exam. Look for abnormally small and cramped handwriting.
    - *Tremor:* Observe the patient's hands while resting. Look for a resting tremor, typically described as "pill-rolling." Tremors may diminish with voluntary movement.

Suggestive clinical features

Severe neuroleptic sensitivity: Adverse reactions to typical antipsychotic medications and high-potency second-generation antipsychotics, like risperidone. Even one dose of a high-potency neuroleptic can impair movement for months and increase mortality in people with DLB/PDD.

CASE VIGNETTE 3: *Mrs. Hernandez, a 79-year-old retired physicist diagnosed with DLB, was prescribed risperidone for hallucinations. Within a week, she developed severe rigidity, confusion, and a marked decline in her overall condition. She discontinued the medication and switched to a low dose of quetiapine. This resulted in some but not total improvement.*

Indicative biomarkers

- *Reduced dopamine transporter uptake in the basal ganglia demonstrated by SPECT or PET:* Helps to distinguish DLB from AD. Reduced dopamine transporter uptake in the basal ganglia is consistent with parkinsonism. It is otherwise nonspecific and rarely ordered.
- *Polysomnographic confirmation of REM sleep without atonia* establishes the diagnosis of RBD.

Diagnostic Criteria from the DLB Consortium

Probable DLB can be diagnosed if

- Criteria are met for dementia.
- There is a subtle and slow progression.
- Two or more core clinical features of DLB are found, with/without biomarkers, or there is just one core clinical feature but with one or more biomarkers (McKeith IG et al, *Neurology* 2017;89(1):88-100).

Differential Diagnosis

DLB vs AD

- *Onset:* DLB has earlier onset of hallucinations and parkinsonism. These occur later in patients with AD.
- *Cognitive fluctuations:* More prominent in DLB than AD.
- *Neurocognitive testing:* Patients with DLB do worse with executive and visuospatial function tasks but do better with memory and naming tests than patients with AD (Galvin JE, *Pract Neurol* 2019;15(5):67-71).
- *Neuroimaging:* There is less pronounced hippocampal atrophy in DLB compared to AD.

DLB vs PDD

- *Timing*
  - DLB is diagnosed if dementia occurs within one year of parkinsonism onset.
  - PDD is diagnosed if dementia develops more than one year after parkinsonism onset.

Table 28: **Differential Diagnosis of Dementia with Lewy Bodies**

Feature	Alzheimer's Dementia (AD)	Dementia with Lewy Bodies (DLB)	Delirium	Parkinson's Disease Dementia (PDD)
Age of Onset	>65 years	>60 years	Any age	>60 years
Onset	Gradual	Gradual; within one year of parkinsonism	Acute/subacute and in the context of active medical illness	Gradual, more than one year after diagnosis of Parkinson's disease
Memory Impairment	Early, short-term memory	Mild initial, progressive	Variable	Mild initial, progressive
Cognitive Fluctuations	Absent or mild	Prominent	Prominent	Present
Parkinsonism	Late, rigidity	Early, mild tremor	Can be present	Early, severe tremor
REM Sleep Behavior Disorder	Rare	Common	Rare	Common
Sensitivity to High-Potency Antipsychotics	Moderate	High	Moderate	High
Visual Hallucinations	Rare (late)	Common (early)	Common	Common (late)
Imaging	Hippocampal and parietal lobe atrophy	Reduced basal ganglia dopamine uptake, less hippocampal atrophy	Typically, normal	Reduced basal ganglia dopamine uptake
Course	Progressive	Progressive	Reversible	Progressive

Dementia with Lewy Bodies: Treatment

Dementia with Lewy Bodies (DLB) is a progressive neurodegenerative disorder characterized by the presence of Lewy bodies in the brain. DLB is the second most common type of progressive dementia after Alzheimer's dementia (AD). This fact sheet will provide practical, evidence-based recommendations for the treatment of DLB, focusing on older adults.

Nonpharmacological Supportive Care

- Refer to an elder care attorney to complete a power of attorney for health care, finances, and advance directives.
- If there is concern about driving ability, complete an on-the-road driving evaluation. Driving can be impacted early in DLB due to executive dysfunction and visuospatial impairments. Hallucinations can also complicate driving.
- Counsel regarding gun safety. This is important for patients who are experiencing paranoia, presence or passage hallucinations, or phantom border delusions. Gun safety might involve removing firearms or placing them in a gun locker/safe to which the patient does not have access.
- Utilize cognitive training programs, such as word searches, crossword puzzles, book clubs, discussion groups, or formal programs, such as Stronger Memory, available at no cost at https://goodwinliving.org/stronger-memory/.
- Physical therapy or occupational therapy assessments should be sought for fall reduction, balance problems, and home safety evaluations for adaptive equipment, such as shower chairs or grab bars.
- Older adult exercise groups, such as Silver Sneakers, Rock Steady Boxing (https://rocksteadyboxing.org), or walking groups, help maintain strength and balance and increase socialization.
- Speech therapy can help with soft speech (hypophonia) and swallowing difficulties (dysphagia).
- Recommend the Mediterranean-DASH Intervention for Neurodegenerative Delay (MIND) diet to optimize heart and brain health.
- Most caregivers will benefit from referral to local LBD educational or support resources (https://www.lbda.org/).

Pharmacological Interventions

Cognitive symptoms

- *Cholinesterase inhibitors*
  - Donepezil
    - Dose: Start at 5 mg daily, increase to 10 mg daily after 4 weeks.
    - Efficacy: Helps stabilize cognition and level of function, though effects are modest and temporary. Cholinesterase inhibitors can also reduce visual hallucinations in people with DLB.
    - Side effects: Nausea, diarrhea, insomnia, weight loss, falls (rare).
  - Rivastigmine
    - Dose: Oral—Start at 1.5 mg twice daily, gradually increasing to 6 mg twice daily. Patch—Start with 4.6 mg/24 hours, increasing to 9.5 mg/24 hours after 4 weeks.
    - Efficacy: Similar to donepezil, with potential additional benefits for behavioral disturbances.
    - Side effects: Gastrointestinal symptoms (fewer with patch), application site reactions (patch), weight loss, falls (rare).

Parkinsonism

Levodopa can be started at 100/25 mg (levodopa/carbidopa) once daily and titrated up to 100/25 mg three times daily. Levodopa may worsen psychosis, including hallucinations. Levodopa is initiated only when the patient has a significant functional impairment, such as difficulty getting out of a car or off a toilet. In most cases, I will defer the management of parkinsonian symptoms to a neurologist.

Hallucinations and delusions

- The goal of treatment is often not to eliminate hallucinations but to make them less frightening and functionally impairing. The first-line treatment is a cholinesterase inhibitor. Second-generation antipsychotics (SGAs) are a second-line option.
- *SGAs* (use with caution due to risk of increased mortality in patients with dementia)
  - Quetiapine
    - Dose: Start at 12.5–25 mg at bedtime, titrate cautiously based on response.
    - Efficacy: May reduce psychotic symptoms with a lower risk of extrapyramidal symptoms.
    - Side effects: Sedation, orthostatic hypotension, QTc prolongation.
  - Pimavanserin
    - Overview: A selective serotonin inverse agonist and antagonist at 5-HT2A receptors. It is FDA-approved for Parkinson's disease psychosis (PDP) but not specifically for DLB. Since it does not target dopamine receptors, it is the least likely to impact movement in patients with DLB/PDP.

- Dose: 34 mg once daily. Adjustments may be necessary based on tolerability and clinical response.
    - Efficacy: First-line choice for PDP; moderate efficacy in reducing neuropsychiatric symptoms. Equally effective to quetiapine for the treatment of hallucinations, but much better tolerated (Horn S and Dahodwala N, *Neurology* 2019;92(15,supplement):P2.8-037).
    - Side effects: Nausea, constipation, less sedation, QTc prolongation, extrapyramidal symptoms (fewer than other antipsychotics).
  - Clozapine
    - Dose: Start at 6.25–12.5 mg at bedtime, titrate slowly and cautiously.
    - Efficacy: Effective for severe psychosis. While it is the drug of choice to treat psychosis in patients with DLB or Parkinson's disease dementia (PDD), increased monitoring and safety concerns keep it as a last resort option.
    - Side effects: Agranulocytosis (requires regular blood monitoring), sedation, orthostatic hypotension, severe constipation, myocarditis, QTc prolongation, and seizures at higher doses.

CASE VIGNETTE 1: *Mr. Thomas, an 80-year-old retired electrician with DLB, experiences significant visual hallucinations and delusions. Quetiapine 25 mg at bedtime is started to help control the symptoms but causes excessive sedation. He is switched to pimavanserin 34 mg daily, which controls the hallucinations with less drowsiness.*

REM sleep behavior disorder (RBD)

- *Melatonin*
  - Dose: Start at 3 mg at bedtime, increase to 6–12 mg based on response.
  - Efficacy: Reduces dream enactment behaviors.
  - Side effects: Rare, may include daytime drowsiness.
- *Clonazepam*
  - Dose: Start at 0.25 mg at bedtime, increase to 0.5–1 mg based on response.
  - Efficacy: Effective for reducing RBD symptoms. RBD is one of the few disorders in older adults in which benzodiazepines are a top-line choice.
  - Side effects: Sedation, increased risk of falls.

CASE VINGETTE 2: *Mr. Johansen, a 75-year-old retired truck driver, experiences vivid dreams and enacts them during sleep. On one occasion, he kicked his wife while dreaming she was an intruder. Melatonin 3 mg at bedtime helps to reduce these episodes. After one month, clonazepam 0.25 mg is added for lingering symptoms, which further improves his sleep with minimal side effects.*

Table 29: **Medications for Dementia with Lewy Bodies**

Medication	Starting Dose	Maximum Dose	Common Side Effects
Clonazepam	0.25 mg at bedtime	1 mg at bedtime	Fall risk, sedation
Clozapine	6.25–12.5 mg at bedtime	Individualized	Agranulocytosis, sedation
Donepezil	5 mg daily	10 mg daily	Diarrhea, insomnia, nausea
Levodopa	100/25 mg once daily	100/25 mg three times daily	Hallucinations, hypotension, nausea
Melatonin	3 mg at bedtime	12 mg at bedtime	Daytime drowsiness
Pimavanserin	34 mg once daily	Individualized	Constipation, nausea
Quetiapine	12.5–25 mg at bedtime	Individualized	Hypotension, sedation
Rivastigmine	1.5 mg twice daily	6 mg twice daily	Gastrointestinal symptoms

Frontotemporal Dementia: Diagnosis

Frontotemporal dementia (FTD) is a group of neurodegenerative disorders characterized by progressive atrophy of the frontal and temporal lobes. It typically affects individuals aged 45–65 but can also present in older adults. It is the second most common dementia, behind Alzheimer's dementia (AD) in people under 65. While most clinicians are familiar with the behavioral variant subtype of FTD, there are a few other subtypes.

Subtypes of FTD

Behavioral variant FTD (bvFTD)

> **CASE VIGNETTE 1:** *Mrs. Alvarez, a 58-year-old former schoolteacher, is brought to the clinic by her family. They report significant personality changes over the past year. She was terminated from her teaching position due to disorganized lectures and occasional cursing in front of her students. In the office, she appears nonplussed. Neuropsychological testing reveals significant deficits in executive functioning but fair memory and visuospatial skills.*

- *Assessment:* Many people with bvFTD will have a poor appreciation of their symptoms, including inappropriate behaviors and changes in personality. Therefore, it is essential to gather history from a knowledgeable collateral informant.
- *Diagnostic criteria*
  - At least three of the following symptoms:
    - Early behavioral disinhibition consisting of socially inappropriate behavior or loss of manners. This can entail inappropriate or offensive comments, nonconsensual touching, and sexual behavior.
      - "Have people noticed any changes in the patient's behavior, such as inappropriate or offensive comments and actions?"
    - Early onset of apathy, inactivity, or indifference.
      - "Has the patient seemed indifferent or unconcerned about things that used to matter to them?"
    - Early loss of empathy toward other people's feelings and needs and diminished social interest.
      - "Has the patient become less responsive to the emotions or problems of family members and friends?"
    - Perseverative or stereotyped behavior that includes repetitive movements, rituals, or compulsions.
    - Hyperorality and dietary changes that consist of binge eating, carbohydrate craving, or mouthing/eating nonfoods.
      - "Has the patient experienced any changes in their eating habits, such as an increased craving for sweets or carbs?"
      - "Do they tend to put things in their mouth that aren't food?"
    - Neuropsychological profile is of executive dysfunction with intact memory and visuospatial skills.
  - For probable bvFTD, there must also be:
    - Criteria met for major neurocognitive disorder (dementia).
    - Subtle and slow progression.
    - Frontal and/or anterior temporal atrophy on MRI/CT or frontal and/or anterior temporal hypoperfusion or hypometabolism on PET/SPECT (Rascovsky K et al, *Brain* 2011;134(9):2456–2477).

Semantic dementia (SD)

> **CASE VIGNETTE 2:** *Mr. Bluth, a 62-year-old former accountant, presents with language difficulties. He struggles to find the right words for things and often uses generic terms like "thing" or "stuff" instead of specific names. Despite this, his memory of recent events and his ability to find his way remain intact. When shown a pen, for the Mini-Mental State Exam, he cannot name it or describe its use. MRI shows atrophy in the anterior temporal lobes.*

- *Clinical features*
  - Language impairment
    - Loss of memory for words or word meaning, leading to difficulty naming and understanding words.
      - "Do you have trouble finding the right words when speaking, even if you know what you want to say?"

Neurocognitive Disorders

        - "Do you sometimes struggle to understand the meaning of words you used to know?"
    - Fluency and grammar are preserved.
    - Speech is empty, with frequent filler or vague words, like "this" or "that."
        - "Do you use more general terms like "thing" or "stuff" because you can't recall the specific word you're looking for?"
  - Cognition: Preserved memory and visuospatial skills.
  - Behavioral features: Disinhibition, impaired judgment.
- *Diagnostic criteria*
  - Progressive loss of word meaning and naming objects.
  - Difficulty in reading and writing.
  - Intact repetition and grammar (Taylor R and Finger E, *Pract Neurol* 2019;15(5);72-77).

Nonfluent primary progressive aphasia (nfPPA)

> **CASE VIGNETTE 3:** *Mrs. Manning, a 70-year-old retired lawyer, has increasing difficulty with her speech. She speaks in short, effortful sentences, often omitting small words and connector words like "and." Her comprehension is relatively preserved, and she can follow complex commands. Imaging reveals atrophy in the left posterior frontal lobe.*

- *Clinical features*
  - Language impairment
    - Effortful, halting speech characterized by slow, labored production.
        - "Have you noticed that speaking has become more difficult, requiring more effort than before?"
        - "Have others mentioned that your speech seems labored or that it takes you longer to express yourself?"
    - Agrammatism and phonemic paraphasias, such as substituting, adding, or rearranging sounds in words (eg, saying "bat" instead of "cat"), are common. As the disease progresses, many patients develop mutism.
        - "Have you had trouble forming complete sentences, instead speaking in short phrases?"
    - Retained word comprehension and naming.
  - Cognition: Preserved memory and visuospatial skills.
  - Behavioral changes: Similar to those experienced by patients with bvFTD but occurring later in the disease course.
- *Diagnostic criteria*
  - One core feature
    - Agrammatism.
    - Effortful speech with inconsistent errors.
  - Two of the following
    - Impaired comprehension of complex sentences.
    - Preserved single-word comprehension.
    - Preserved object knowledge (Taylor R and Finger E 2019).

Differential Diagnosis

AD vs FTD

- AD typically presents later (>65 years) compared to FTD (45-65 years).
- Early and prominent memory impairment is characteristic of AD. In contrast, FTD patients often have relatively preserved memory in the early stages.
- FTD is marked by pronounced personality and behavioral changes, such as disinhibition, apathy, and loss of empathy. AD patients usually show fewer behavioral changes early on and maintain social graces until later in the disease.
- On cognitive testing, patients with FTD score well on short-term recall and orientation but lower on executive function tests, such as clock drawing, and language subtests, like naming or repeating sentences, compared to AD patients.
- MRI or PET scans typically show frontal and anterior temporal lobe atrophy/hypometabolism in bvFTD and medial temporal-parietal atrophy/hypometabolism in AD.

FTD vs primary psychiatric disorders

Psychiatric misdiagnoses occur in up to 50% of bvFTD patients. Careful history taking with strict adherence to diagnostic criteria; neuropsychological testing with a focus on executive function and social cognition; brain MRI or PET scans; and genetic testing help with the differential diagnosis (Ducharme S et al, *Brain* 2020;143(7):1632-1650).

- *Bipolar disorder (BD):* FTD can be misdiagnosed as BD due to overlapping symptoms like disinhibition, hypersexuality, risky behaviors, and mood changes. Patients in the throes of a manic episode may also score poorly on cognitive testing due to difficulty sustaining focus and attention. However, patients who are manic typically have elated moods with increased energy symptoms, like decreased need for sleep, rapid speech, and increased goal-directed activity. These are not common features of bvFTD. Patients who are manic will also return to baseline once the mood episode has resolved, while bvFTD is a chronic and progressive disease.
- *Schizophrenia:* FTD can present occasionally with psychosis-like symptoms, such as hallucinations and delusions, leading to a misdiagnosis of schizophrenia. People with schizophrenia usually have more pronounced psychotic features, particularly paranoia in late life, without the prominent executive dysfunction seen in patients with FTD.

Table 30: **Differentiation of Frontotemporal Dementia, Alzheimer's Dementia, and Other Disorders**

Feature	bvFTD	SD	nfPPA	AD	Acute Mania	Acute Psychosis
Onset	Earlier (45-65 years)	Earlier (45-65 years)	Earlier (45-65 years)	Later (>65 years)	Any age	Any age
Memory	Relatively preserved initially	Preserved memory	Preserved memory	Early and prominent short-term memory impairment	Typically preserved but may score poorly on tests	Typically preserved but may score poorly on tests
Behavior	Significant changes, disinhibition	Similar to bvFTD but less pronounced	Similar to bvFTD but more prominent changes in later stages	Less prominent changes early on	Elevated mood, grandiosity, disinhibition	Paranoia, delusions, hallucinations
Language	Variable, less prominent	Loss of word meaning	Effortful, halting speech	Less prominent deficits early on	Pressured speech, flight of ideas	Disorganized speech
Visuospatial Skills	Preserved in early stages	Preserved	Preserved	Impaired	Preserved	Preserved
Imaging	Frontal lobe atrophy	Anterior temporal lobe atrophy, left > right	Left posterior frontoinsular atrophy	Medial temporal and parietal lobe atrophy	White matter hyperintensities	Normal or subcortical abnormalities
Genetic Testing	Commonly associated genes in 40%-50% are GRN, C9orf72, MAPT	Sporadic	Associated genes: GRN, C9orf72	Associated genes: APOE ε4, PSEN1, PSEN2, APP	Not applicable	Not applicable

Frontotemporal Dementia: Treatment

Frontotemporal dementia (FTD) encompasses a group of neurodegenerative disorders that primarily affect the frontal and temporal lobes of the brain, leading to progressive changes in behavior, personality, and language. Treatment strategies for FTD focus on managing symptoms, as no FDA-approved therapies exist. The best evidence for neuropsychiatric symptoms (NPS) due to FTD is for citalopram and trazodone. See the fact sheet "Frontotemporal Dementia: Diagnosis" [page 115] for tips on identifying FTD in older adults.

Nonpharmacological Treatments

Implement legal and safety measures

- ***Establish power of attorney:*** Ensure a power of attorney for health care and finances is in place to manage risks related to poor judgment, impulsive behavior, and spending. Since people with FTD are mostly younger, this is a critical step to protect the patient's assets and interests.
- ***Assess driving safety:*** Evaluate the patient's driving abilities with an on-the-road driving evaluation. Patients with FTD struggle with attention, complex road conditions, and impulsivity, increasing the risk of accidents.
- ***Advice regarding firearm safety:*** Recommend that caregivers remove firearms from the home or securely store them in a gun safe that the patient cannot access to prevent accidents.

CASE VIGNETTE 1: *Mr. Patrick, a 63-year-old man with behavioral variant frontotemporal dementia (bvFTD), displays impulsive and disinhibited behavior, including verbal aggression toward family members. Mr. Patrick has always been an avid gun owner, and his wife is concerned about the presence of firearms in the home. Due to the risk of impulsivity and potential harm, his family is advised to remove firearms from the home or lock them securely in a safe to which Mr. Patrick has no access. With the implementation of this last safety measure, his family begins to feel more secure.*

Enhance communication

Use speech therapy to help maintain language skills or facilitate communication through alternative methods such as communication books or assistive technology. This is especially crucial for patients with semantic dementia and nonfluent primary progressive aphasia (nfPPA).

Promote physical and cognitive activities

- ***Encourage regular exercise:*** Promote regular aerobic exercise to improve strength and balance, reduce fall risk, and slow disease progression.
- ***Stimulate cognition:*** Engage patients in regular cognitive activities to slow the rate of cognitive decline and reduce disease severity.

Use occupational therapy strategies

Optimize daily function: Occupational therapists can assess cognitive and physical status and provide strategies like step-by-step activity guides with pictures for tasks like computer or cell phone logins to support patients with executive dysfunction.

Prevent choking

Monitor eating habits: Have caregivers supervise patients during meals to prevent choking, particularly if the patient eats quickly, overfills their mouth, or attempts to eat nonfood items. Advise caregivers to offer reduced, more frequent portions or smaller bites to mitigate risk.

CASE VIGNETTE 2: *Mr. Iverson, a 58-year-old man diagnosed with behavioral variant frontotemporal dementia (bvFTD), exhibits compulsive eating behaviors with a preference for sweets. These behaviors are characterized by rapid consumption, increasing the risk of choking incidents. Additionally, nocturnal snacking is observed, further exacerbating the risk and contributing to weight gain. To address these challenges, sertraline is started at 25 mg daily. Concurrently, his family implements safety measures by securing cabinets and the refrigerator to prevent unsupervised access to food. To provide alternatives, they leave out healthy finger-foods that can be consumed safely.*

Support caregivers

Direct caregivers to dementia help groups, such as the Association for Frontotemporal Deterioration (AFTD) at www.aftd.org, for resources and emotional support.

CASE VIGNETTE 3: *Ms. Lalitha, a 65-year-old woman with bvFTD, exhibits inappropriate behaviors (eg, walking up to strangers and making offensive comments). She has had episodes of unprovoked aggression, including yelling at her family members and throwing objects during meals. Her psychiatrist initiates and titrates escitalopram to 20 mg/day. This partially improves her symptoms. Next, quetiapine 25 mg qHS is added. This is eventually titrated to 100 mg qHS. Over the following months, Ms. Lalitha's aggression and inappropriate behaviors diminish, significantly improving her interactions with others.*

Antidepressants

FTD significantly disrupts the action of serotonin in the frontal lobes. This causes many of its classic symptoms, including disinhibition, impulsivity, repetitive behaviors, eating concerns, and behavioral dysregulation. The primary treatment for behaviors due to FTD are serotonergic antidepressants.

- *Selective serotonin reuptake inhibitors (SSRIs)*
  - *Indications:* Used to manage many types of FTD behavioral disturbances.
  - *Efficacy:* The best evidence is for citalopram. Given the potential for QTc prolongation with citalopram, escitalopram is a reasonable alternative.
  - *Medications and dosages:*
    - Citalopram: Start at 10 mg/day, titrate to 20 mg/day, the FDA maximum in older adults.
    - Escitalopram: Start at 5 mg/day, titrate to 20 mg/day.
    - Sertraline: Start at 25 mg/day, titrate to 50–200 mg/day.
    - Fluvoxamine: Start at 25 mg/day, titrate to 50–150 mg/day. Fluvoxamine may be effective for OCD-like symptoms when other antidepressants have failed.
- *Serotonin norepinephrine reuptake inhibitors (SNRIs)*
  - *Indications:* Can be helpful for managing co-occurring depression and anxiety.
  - *Medications and dosages*
    - Venlafaxine: Start at 37.5 mg/day, titrate to 75–225 mg/day.
    - Duloxetine: Start at 30 mg/day, titrate to 60–90 mg/day.
- *Trazodone*
  - *Indications:* Trazodone has been effective in treating agitation, irritability, depression, and aggression in FTD (Lebert F et al, *Dement Geriatr Cogn Disord* 2004;17(4):355-359).
  - *Dosages:* Start at 25 mg at bedtime, titrate to 50–300 mg at bedtime or in divided doses.

Second-generation antipsychotics (SGAs)

- *Indications:* SGAs may be helpful for severe agitation, psychosis, and disinhibition in FTD. However, given the risk of parkinsonism and motor neuron disease in FTD patients, lower-potency agents are preferred. Antipsychotics should be used cautiously due to increased mortality risk in patients with dementia.
- *Medications and dosages*
  - Quetiapine: Favored due to lower risk of extrapyramidal symptoms. Start at 25 mg/day, titrate to 100–300 mg/day as needed.
  - Aripiprazole: Start at 2 mg/day, titrate to 5–15 mg/day.
  - Olanzapine: Start at 2.5 mg/day, titrate to 5–10 mg/day.

Mood stabilizers

- *Indications:* May help with mood swings, impulsivity, and aggressive behaviors.
- *Medications and dosages*
  - Lithium: Start at 150 mg/day, titrate to 600 mg/day. Aim for serum levels of 0.2–0.6 mmol/L
  - Valproic acid: Start at 250 mg/day, titrate to 500–1000 mg/day.
  - Carbamazepine: Start at 100 mg/day, titrate to 200–600 mg/day.

Medications to avoid

- *Acetylcholinesterase inhibitors* can potentially worsen cognitive and neuropsychiatric symptoms in individuals with FTD. However, this may not apply to patients with nfPPA, as a significant proportion of this population (up to 40%) has underlying AD pathology (Taylor R and Finger E, *Pract Neurol* 2019;15(5):72–77).
- *High-potency antipsychotics* may increase mortality and have a high incidence of motor side effects.
- *Memantine* has shown no benefit and may worsen cognition in people with FTD.

Table 31: **Pharmacological Treatments for Frontotemporal Dementia**

Medication Type	Medication	Indication	Starting Dose	Maintenance Dose
SSRIs	Citalopram	Agitation, anxiety, compulsions, depression, disinhibition, disordered eating, impulsivity, stereotyped movements	10 mg/day	10–20 mg/day
	Escitalopram	Agitation, anxiety, compulsions, depression, disinhibition, disordered eating, impulsivity, stereotyped movements	5 mg/day	10–20 mg/day
	Fluvoxamine	Compulsions, OCD, stereotyped movements	25 mg/day	50–150 mg/day
	Sertraline	Agitation, anxiety, compulsions, depression, disinhibition, disordered eating, impulsivity, stereotyped movements	25 mg/day	50–200 mg/day
SNRIs	Duloxetine	Depression, anxiety	30 mg/day	60–120 mg/day
	Venlafaxine	Depression, anxiety	37.5 mg/day	75–225 mg/day
Other Antidepressants	Trazodone	Aggression, agitation, depression, insomnia, irritability	25 mg/qhs	50–300 mg/qhs or in divided doses (BID or TID)
Second-generation Antipsychotics	Aripiprazole	Severe agitation, psychosis	2 mg/day	5–15 mg/day
	Olanzapine	Severe agitation, psychosis	2.5 mg/day	5–10 mg/day
	Quetiapine	Severe agitation, psychosis	25 mg/day	100–300 mg/day
Mood Stabilizers	Carbamazepine	Impulsivity, mood swings	100 mg/day	200–600 mg/day
	Lithium	Aggression, impulsivity, mood swings	150 mg/qhs	150–600 mg/qhs; maintain serum levels 0.2–0.6 mmol/L
	Valproic Acid	Aggression, impulsivity, mood swings	250 mg/day	500–1000 mg/day

Vascular Dementia: Diagnosis and Treatment

Vascular dementia (VaD) is caused by cerebrovascular compromise, most frequently as the result of strokes. It is the second most prevalent type of dementia, accounting for approximately 15%–20% of cases. Risk factors include hypertension, diabetes, hyperlipidemia, smoking, atrial fibrillation, and other cardiovascular diseases.

Pathophysiology

- Cerebrovascular damage can occur from wide-ranging etiologies. These involve:
  - Small vessel disease: This is the primary cause in most cases and leads to white matter lesions and lacunar infarcts.
  - Large vessel infarctions: These strokes impact larger brain regions.
  - Genetics: CADASIL (cerebral autosomal dominant arteriopathy with subcortical infarcts and leukoencephalopathy) is the most common inherited cause of VaD.
- Damage to cerebrovasculature can be caused by single, multiple, or diffuse injuries.
- Mixed dementia: VaD often coexists with Alzheimer's dementia (AD), complicating diagnosis and treatment.

DSM-5-TR Criteria for Major Vascular Neurocognitive Disorder

- Evidence of substantial cognitive decline from an earlier level of performance.
- There is decline in attention, processing speed, and executive function.
- There is confirmed cerebrovascular disease from history, physical examination, or neuroimaging, which is enough to explain the deficits.
- The cognitive deficits hamper independence in everyday activities.
- At least one of the following is present:
  - Neuroimaging evidence of cerebrovascular damage.
  - An association in time between cerebrovascular events and cognitive decline.
  - Clinical and genetic evidence of cerebrovascular disease, such as from CADASIL.

Clinical Presentation

Cognitive symptoms

- Stepwise deterioration in cognitive function is the classic description, but it is often difficult to elicit from patients and caregivers.
- Ask about:
  - Sudden and lasting changes in cognitive abilities following strokes or transient ischemic attacks.
  - Any periods of relatively stable memory followed by sudden declines.
- Impairment in executive function and slowed processing speed are early findings. On the Montreal Cognitive Assessment (MoCA), this might result in difficulty connecting numbers to letters in sequence (trail-making test) or drawing a clock with the hands placed correctly.
- Working memory, which involves holding and manipulating information in memory, is also impacted. This can manifest on the MoCA as difficulty with backward digit span, counting backwards by 7s from 100, letter fluency, or sentence repetition.
- People with VaD may struggle with attention and multitasking (ie, dividing attention). On the MoCA, patients may also have trouble with the forward and backward digit span, the serial sevens, and the letter A tap.

Behavioral and psychological symptoms

- People with VaD have high rates of depression and apathy.
- Less common are hallucinations and delusions.

CASE VIGNETTE 1: *After a stroke, Mr. Singh, an 80-year-old man, suddenly has trouble organizing his daily tasks and paying bills. He is easily distracted and has trouble following complex instructions, although his memory remains fair.*

CASE VIGNETTE 2: *Mrs. Ali, a 75-year-old woman, shows a gradual decline in her ability to manage her medication and finances. Her daughter notices she has become increasingly apathetic, often withdrawing from family activities. MRI reveals significant white matter changes indicative of extensive small vessel disease.*

Differential Diagnosis

Alzheimer's disease

AD presents with early memory loss. The Hachinski Ischemic Scale (Hachinski VC et al, *Arch Neurol 1975*;32(9):632-637) can help differentiate VaD from AD. Points are assigned based on clinical features, with a higher score indicating a greater likelihood of VaD. Some indicators of VaD are sudden onset, stepwise progression, fluctuating course, history of strokes, focal neurological symptoms, and focal neurological signs.

Table 32: **Key Differences Between Alzheimer's Dementia and Vascular Dementia**

Feature	Alzheimer's Dementia	Vascular Dementia
Onset	Gradual	Sudden or stepwise
Cognitive Symptoms	Language deficits, short-term memory loss, visuospatial impairment	Executive dysfunction, impaired attention
Course	Progressive	Fluctuating
Neuroimaging	Hippocampal and parietal lobe atrophy	Infarcts, microhemorrhages, white matter hyperintensities
Risk Factors	Age, family history	Diabetes, hypertension, stroke

Treatment

Nonpharmacological interventions

- *Lifestyle modification*
  - There are no FDA-approved medications for VaD, so the primary treatment is to reduce the risk of further cerebrovascular damage. Usually, this will be managed by the patient's PCP, cardiologist, or stroke neurologist.
  - Elements to emphasize:
    - Regulate cardiovascular risk factors (eg, hypertension, diabetes, sleep apnea, hyperlipidemia, atrial fibrillation, and homocysteinemia).
      - To encourage adherence to treatment, I tell patients, "Heart health is brain health," and "The healthier your heart is, the healthier your brain will be."
    - Smoking cessation and reduction of alcohol intake.
    - Regular physical exercise and a balanced diet.
- *Cognitive rehabilitation*
  - Focuses on memory (spaced repetition, memory aids), executive function (planning, problem-solving), attention (dual-task exercises), language (storytelling, word-finding), and visuospatial skills (puzzles, navigation).
  - Recovery from a stroke can take a year or longer, so this should be a sustained effort.
- *Occupational therapy*
  - Enhances daily living skills (cooking, dressing) and ensures safety with home modifications and assistive devices (pill organizers, grab bars) based on physical and cognitive limitations.
- *Caregiver support*
  - Inform caregivers about the nature of the disease and its progression.
  - Provide support and referral to support groups or mental health treatment as needed.
- *Advance care planning:* Encourage discussions about creating a power of attorney and advance directives.

Pharmacological treatment

- *Acetylcholinesterase inhibitors (Donepezil, Galantamine, Rivastigmine)*
  - Are used off-label with largely modest benefits in cognitive function and daily activities.
  - Donepezil 10 mg and galantamine 16–24 mg positively affect cognition in people with VaD. Rivastigmine in small trials was not helpful (Battle CE et al, *Cochrane Database Syst Rev* 2021;2(2):CD013306).
- *Memantine*
  - Has been prescribed off-label with limited benefit (O'Brien JT and Thomas A, *Lancet 2015*;386(10004):1698-706).
  - It may be considered, along with cholinesterase inhibitors, in patients who have moderate to severe mixed dementia with significant AD pathology.
- *Comorbid conditions*
  - Depression: Selective serotonin reuptake inhibitors (SSRIs) or serotonin-norepinephrine reuptake inhibitors (SNRIs) may be helpful. If the patient has significant neurovegetative symptoms or apathy, consider bupropion or augmenting with a stimulant, such as methylphenidate or modafinil.
  - Anxiety: Nonbenzodiazepine anxiolytics such as SSRIs, SNRIs, buspirone, or gabapentin are preferred due to their lower risk of cognitive side effects.

Cognitive Enhancers for Dementia

Cognitive enhancers slow down memory loss but do not stop or reverse dementia. They are most effective for Alzheimer's dementia (AD), dementia with Lewy bodies (DLB), and Parkinson's disease dementia (PDD). Once a patient is diagnosed with one of these dementias, start a cognitive enhancer right away.

Choosing a Cognitive Enhancer for Dementia

Acetylcholinesterase inhibitors (AChEI)

- *Donepezil*
  - First-line treatment for most patients with AD.
  - Usually, well tolerated but may cause gastrointestinal (GI) side effects in 20% of people, including nausea, vomiting, and diarrhea. Switch to the rivastigmine transdermal patch if GI side effects do not resolve.
- *Rivastigmine*
  - Oral formulation
    - First-line choice for patients with DLB or PDD.
    - Switch to the transdermal patch if GI side effects occur.
  - Patch formulation
    - Preferred in patients who are unable to tolerate oral AChEIs due to GI side effects, as it is associated with a lower rate of GI disturbances.
    - Offers convenient dosing and better adherence in some patients.
    - Counsel patients and families to apply the patch to clean, dry, hairless skin on the back, upper arm, or chest and to rotate sites daily to prevent skin irritation.
- *Galantamine*
  - Third-line option for AD due to a less favorable side effect profile and limited evidence compared to donepezil and rivastigmine.
  - May have a specific role in vascular dementia, though evidence is modest.
- *Efficacy of AChEIs*
  - AChEIs slow down memory decline for approximately 6 months in most patients.
  - They may delay the onset of behavioral and psychological symptoms of dementia (BPSD) if started early.

Memantine

- *Indication and use*
  - Initiate when patients reach the moderate stage of dementia and continue it to the severe stage of dementia.
  - Often combined with an AChEI for synergistic benefit.
- *Efficacy*
  - When used in combination with an AChEI, memory loss may be slowed by up to 9 months.
  - Modest impact on reducing BPSD, especially agitation.

Recommendations

- *Early initiation*
  - Start cognitive enhancers as soon as possible after diagnosing dementia to maximize benefits.
  - Titrate to the highest tolerated dose.
  - Continue therapy through moderate and severe stages unless significant functional decline warrants discontinuation.
- *Patient-specific choice*
  - Tailor selection based on dementia subtype and tolerance:
    - AD: Donepezil is first-line; switch to rivastigmine patch if GI intolerance occurs.
    - DLB/PDD: Start with oral rivastigmine; switch to the patch if GI side effects occur.
    - Vascular dementia: Could trial galantamine, which can also be considered for other dementia subtypes if other agents are unable to be tolerated. Another choice is donepezil.
- *Counseling families*
  - Set realistic expectations:
    - Emphasize that cognitive enhancers modestly slow memory decline but do not reverse or halt disease progression.
    - Inform families that benefits may not be overtly noticeable, but the medicine may help prevent sudden declines or BPSD, as well as delay nursing home placement.

- Highlight risks of stopping treatment prematurely:
  - Patients may experience a rapid decline to a lower baseline after discontinuation, which will not recover even if the medications are restarted.
- *Combination therapy*
  - Combine memantine with an AChEI in moderate to severe dementia for enhanced benefit on cognition and function.
  - Recommend, due to their modest benefits, ordering medications within the context of a holistic treatment strategy, that also incorporates a healthy diet, physical exercise, socialization, and cognitive stimulation.
- *Discontinuation*
  - Consider stopping medications in advanced dementia when there is significant impairment in basic activities of daily living, such as incontinence, bedbound status, or nonverbal state.

Table 33: **Prescribing Guidelines for Common Dementia Medications**

Medication	Starting Dose	Titration and Max Dose	Formulations	Preferred Use	Monitoring
Donepezil	5 mg/day	Increase to 10 mg/day after 4 weeks; 23 mg/day tablet may cause more side effects with limited additional benefit	Tablet, patch, disintegrating tablet	First-line for most patients	Monitor for diarrhea, nausea, bradycardia, weight loss, and falls
Rivastigmine	1.5 mg BID	Increase by 1.5 mg q2Weeks; max 6 mg BID; transdermal: start at 4.6 mg daily, increase after 4 weeks, max 13.3 mg daily	Capsule, transdermal patch	Preferentially used in patients with PDD or DLB	Monitor for GI side effects, weight loss, falls; transdermal form has fewer GI side effects but may cause rare skin rashes at patch site
Galantamine	4 mg BID	Increase to 8 mg BID after 4 weeks, then to 12 mg BID after 4 weeks	Tablet, extended-release capsule, liquid	Alternative option	Monitor for GI side effects, bradycardia, weight loss, and falls
Memantine	5 mg nightly	Increase weekly by 5 mg/day in divided doses to 10 mg BID	Tablet, extended-release capsule, liquid	Reserved for moderate and severe dementia; combine with an AChEI for best effect	Monitor for dizziness, sedation, confusion; adjust dose for kidney insufficiency

Parkinson's Disease: Psychiatric Aspects

Neuropsychiatric disorders are common in Parkinson's disease (PD), especially in older adults. These disturbances include anxiety, apathy, cognitive impairment, depression, impulse control disorders, psychosis, and sleep disruptions. This fact sheet aims to provide clinicians with an approach to managing neuropsychiatric presentations due to PD.

What is PD?

PD is a progressive neurodegenerative disorder characterized by the loss of dopaminergic neurons in the substantia nigra. It is the second most common neurodegenerative condition in older adults, behind Alzheimer's disease (AD).

Symptoms

- The four main motor symptoms of PD are **TRAP**
  - **T**remor (resting)
  - **R**igidity
  - **A**kinesia (slowed movements)
  - **P**ostural instability (contributes to falls)
- Secondary symptoms include diminished arm swing, decreased blink rate, reduced facial expression (hypomimia), decreased voice volume (hypophonia), and difficulty turning.
- Nonmotor symptoms, such as loss of smell (hyposmia) and constipation, are common and can begin years before the disease.

Etiology

The exact cause is unknown but involves a combination of genetic and environmental factors.

Diagnosis

Primarily clinical, based on motor symptoms and response to dopaminergic therapy. Imaging and laboratory tests can support the diagnosis by ruling out other causes.

Anxiety

Prevalence

Affects up to 40% of patients with PD.

Symptoms

- *Common symptoms*
  - Excessive worry
  - Restlessness
  - Muscle tension
  - Irritability
  - Sleep disturbances
  - Panic attacks
- *PD specific symptoms*
  - Internal tremor is a sense of vibration in the body that is not observable. It can account for anxiety in 64% of patients with PD and often improves with anxiety therapies (Higinbotham AS and Gunzler SA, *Current Psychiatry* 2023;22(10):15-24).
  - Nonmotor "off" anxiety: As levodopa doses wear off, patients may enter an "off" state in which they freeze or their movements slow. The dopamine withdrawal and feeling of being trapped or stuck leads to anxiety and panic.

Treatment (in order of preference)

- *SSRIs*
  - Sertraline: 25–200 mg/day
  - Citalopram: 10–20 mg/day
- *TCAs (watch for arrhythmias, falls, orthostatic hypotension, and QTc prolongation)*
  - Desipramine: 25–100 mg/day (once or divided)
  - Nortriptyline: 25–75 mg/day (divided or at bedtime)
- *Bupropion:* Can be helpful for anxiety related to low dopamine levels.
- *Benzodiazepines (short-term use due to risk of dependence and cognitive impairment):*
  - Clonazepam: 0.25–2 mg/day (can also help with rigidity).
- *Dopaminergic Agents*
  - Levodopa: Increasing the dose might help with general anxiety and also with nonmotor "off" anxiety.

Neurocognitive Disorders

- Ropinirole: 0.25–4 mg/day (can help with restless legs syndrome too but may cause hypotension and compulsive behaviors).
- *Psychotherapy:* Cognitive behavioral therapy (CBT) for anxiety.

Apathy

Prevalence

Affects up to 40% of patients.

Symptoms

- Lack of motivation
- Reduced interest in activities
- Emotional indifference

Clinical questions

- "Do you feel less motivated to engage in activities you once enjoyed?"
- "Have you noticed a lack of interest in social or recreational activities?"
- "Do you feel emotionally flat or indifferent?"

Treatment

- Routine and structure
  - Establish regular daily routines to help patients stay engaged and active.
  - Consider exercise programs such as physical therapy, Silver Sneakers (https://tools.silversneakers.com/), or Rock Steady Boxing (https://www.rocksteadyboxing.org/).
  - Increase social engagement via senior centers or day programs.
- Bupropion: 75–300 mg/day, may help with amotivation.
- Stimulants
  - Atomoxetine: 40 mg/day (potential for QTc prolongation)
  - Methylphenidate: 5–20 mg/day (limited evidence)
- Dopamine agonists
  - Amantadine: 100 mg daily to 100 mg BID (watch for depression, edema, falls, hallucinations, livedo reticularis, orthostatic hypotension)
  - Pramipexole: 0.125 mg three times daily, to 4.5 mg/day (monitor for hallucinations, delusions, impulse control disorders, and dyskinesias)
  - Ropinirole: 0.25 mg three times daily to 3 mg/day (similar adverse reactions as pramipexole)
- Cholinesterase inhibitors, like rivastigmine, can help with apathy.

Cognitive Impairment and Dementia

Prevalence

Mild cognitive impairment (MCI) occurs in 25% and dementia is present in 30%–80% of people with PD (Weintraub D and Mamikonyan E, *Am J Geriatric Psychiatry* 2019;27(9):998–1018).

Symptoms

- Memory problems
- Trouble with attention
- Difficulty with executive function (planning, organizing, sequencing)
- Language struggles
- Visuospatial impairment

Clinical questions

- "Have you had trouble remembering things recently?"
- "Do you find it difficult to plan and organize tasks?"
- "Have you noticed any changes in your ability to find the right words or understand conversations?"

Treatment

- *Cholinesterase inhibitors*
  - Rivastigmine: 1.5–6 mg twice daily (or 4.6–13.3 mg/24 hr patch) (only FDA-approved treatment for PD dementia)
  - Donepezil: 5–10 mg/day
- *NMDA receptor antagonist*:
  - Memantine: 5–20 mg/day (for moderate to severe dementia)

Depression

Prevalence

Affects up to 50% of patients with PD.

Symptoms (compared to non-PD patients with depression)

- Higher anxiety
- Persistent sadness
- Irritability
- More pessimism and negativity
- Suicidal ideation without suicidal behavior
- Less guilt and feelings of worthlessness (Leentjens A, J *Geriatr Psychiatry Neurol* 2004;17(3):120-126)

Treatment (in order of preference)

- *Bupropion*: 75–300 mg/day (useful for addressing co-occurring apathy and amotivation)
- *SNRIs (Serotonin Norepinephrine Reuptake Inhibitors)*
  - Venlafaxine: 37.5–225 mg/day
- *SSRIs (Selective Serotonin Reuptake Inhibitors)*
  - Sertraline: 25–200 mg/day
  - Escitalopram: 10–20 mg/day
  - Paroxetine: 10–40 mg/day (third-line option due to strong anticholinergic effect)
- *Tricyclic antidepressants*
  - Nortriptyline: 25–100 mg/day (consider cardiac side effects, such as QTc prolongation, arrhythmias, orthostatic hypotension, and conduction delays)
- *Psychotherapy*: CBT is beneficial.
- *Electroconvulsive therapy*: Can improve treatment-resistant depression and temporarily PD, by causing a massive dopamine release from neurons.

Impulse Control Disorders

Prevalence

Affects up to 15%–20% of patients.

Etiology

ICDs occur due to hypersensitivity to rewarding behavior or to hyperdopaminergic states brought on by dopamine agonists or levodopa.

Presentations

- *Binge eating*
- *Compulsive buying/shopping*
- *Dopamine dysregulation syndrome (DDRS)*
  - DDRS is associated with dopamine addiction.
  - It typically manifests in younger male patients who have minimal motor symptoms but have dyskinesias.
  - Characteristics include taking increasing doses of levodopa or dopamine agonists beyond what is needed to manage motor symptoms. Medication hoarding, demanding early refills, or exaggerating motor-off states to obtain more medication can also occur.
  - Mood and behavior symptoms include euphoria or hypomania, dysphoria or depression, irritability, aggression, and impulsivity.
- *Hypersexuality*
  - Found in approximately 3.5% of patients, it is more common in those using dopamine agonists.
  - Symptoms include increased preoccupation with sexual thoughts, frequent demands for sex, habitual use of internet pornography, and engaging with sex workers.
- *Pathological gambling*
- *Punding*
  - Excessive and intense preoccupation with items or activities without a clear purpose. It is seen in younger patients. High doses of PD meds can induce it.

Clinical questions

- "Have you noticed any urges or behaviors that are difficult to control?"
- "Have you been spending more money than usual, gambling, or engaging in risky behaviors?"
- "Have there been any changes in your sexual behavior?"

Treatment

- Adjust PD medications: Reduce or discontinue dopamine agonists.
- Cognitive behavioral therapy: To address underlying impulses and behaviors.

- Marshal caregivers to monitor symptoms and limit access to triggers, including dopamine agonists (in people with DDRS), as well as canceling credit cards and blocking access to casinos, gambling websites/apps, or pornography.
- SSRIs: For impulse dyscontrol as well as to manage associated anxiety and depression.
- Antipsychotics: Quetiapine or clozapine for severe cases.

Psychosis

Prevalence

Occurs in up to 50% of patients with PD and is a predictor of mortality, caregiver distress, and nursing home placement. Insight is often preserved, which can help distinguish it from psychotic disorders in which insight is regularly lost.

Common symptoms

- *Hallucinations*
  - Visual: Seeing people, animals, or objects that are not there. Common examples include seeing a person standing in the room, animals like cats or dogs, or people peering through the windows.
  - Passage: Involves the sensation of a person or animal passing in the peripheral visual field.
  - Presence: Feeling that someone is present in the room when in fact no one is there.
  - Tactile: Feeling physical sensations (eg, someone touching or grabbing).
- *Delusions*
  - Capgras: Belief that a familiar person, usually a close family member, has been replaced by an imposter.
  - Othello syndrome: Jealous delusions involving infidelity. Patients may believe their spouse is having an affair whenever they are out of sight.
  - Paranoid: Believing that others are trying to harm the individual or are conspiring against them.
  - Phantom boarder syndrome: False belief that someone is living in or visiting the person's home.
  - Reduplicative paramnesia: Belief that a familiar person, place, or object has been duplicated.

When to treat

- *Hallucinations/delusions with/without insight:* If not distressing or disruptive, they may not require immediate treatment. Monitor the patient regularly.
- *Moderate to severe hallucinations/delusions without insight:* If they cause significant distress, fear, or behavioral changes, then treatment is indicated.
- *Disruptive or dangerous symptoms:* These can lead to risky behaviors, such as wandering, agitation, refusal of care, or aggression toward the "imposter" or partner in the case of jealousy. Immediate treatment is necessary.

Treatment

- *Antipsychotics (use with caution due to potential worsening of motor symptoms)*
  - Quetiapine: 12.5–150 mg/day
  - Pimavanserin (Nuplazid): 34 mg/day
    - Mechanism: Inverse agonist and antagonist at serotonin 5-HT2A receptors. It has no activity at the dopamine receptors, so it is ideal for treating psychosis in patients with PD without worsening motor symptoms.
    - Efficacy: Generally, it takes more than two weeks to show effectiveness.
    - Considerations: It is the only medication FDA-approved for PD psychosis. It is expensive and may not be covered by insurance.
  - Clozapine: 12.5–100 mg/day (requires regular blood monitoring for agranulocytosis)
- *Adjust PD medications*
  - Some PD medications may contribute to psychosis. If symptoms continue despite antipsychotic treatment, discuss with the patient's neurologist and consider recommending reduction or discontinuation of PD medications in this order:
    - Anticholinergics
    - Amantadine
    - Dopamine agonists
    - Selegiline or rasagiline
    - COMT inhibitors
    - Levodopa

Agitation in Dementia: Urgent Treatment

Urgent agitation threatens the safety and well-being of the patient and others, like caregivers and staff. It can take the form of physical aggression, violence toward objects, resistance to care, distressing hallucinations or delusions, or uncontrollable screaming. For rapid relief of symptoms, IMs, IVs, or ODTs are preferred over tablets or capsules, which are absorbed more slowly. These recommendations are partly based on comprehensive algorithms published by Chen A et al (*Psychiatry Research* 2021;295:113641) and Davies SJC et al (*Journal of Psychopharmacology* 2018;32(5):509–523).

Urgent Treatment of Behavioral and Psychological Disturbances in Dementia (BPSD)

Trial medications in the following order:

IM/ODT olanzapine

- 5 mg PO ODT OR 1.25–5 mg IM, may repeat X 3 over 24 hours.
- Maximum total dose over 24 hours is 15 mg.
- Provide doses in at least 30-minute intervals.

IM/IV haloperidol

- 1–2.5 mg IM OR 0.5–1 mg IV.
- Wait at least one hour for response and repeat PRN.
- There is a greater risk of QTc prolongation with IV compared to IM haloperidol.
- First-generation antipsychotics are recommended only for urgent agitation.

IM/IV benzodiazepines

- Order lorazepam 0.5–1 mg IM OR 0.5–1 mg IV q4h, with max dose of 2 mg in 24 hours.
- Benzodiazepines (BZD) are not recommended for nonurgent BPSD due to risks of worsened confusion and falls.
- BZDs cause hypotension if combined with olanzapine; recommend waiting at least one hour following IM olanzapine administration to administer a BZD.
- BZD are preferable to olanzapine or haloperidol for patients with Parkinson's disease dementia, dementia with Lewy bodies, recent neuroleptic malignant syndrome, or patients pending medical procedures.

Last resort

These options are riskier and have little to no research data behind them:

- SL dexmedetomidine
- IM ziprasidone
- IV diazepam
- IM midazolam

Agitation in Dementia: Nonurgent Treatment

Nonurgent agitation consists of distressing symptoms and behaviors that do not immediately jeopardize patient or caregiver safety. Some examples are pacing and fidgeting, resisting care or activities of daily living (ADLs) like bathing, distressed vocalizations, and showing irritability or frustration over minor issues. While we usually choose antipsychotics for urgent agitation, we use them more sparingly for nonurgent agitation due to boxed warnings for an increased risk of stroke and death in patients with dementia with this medication class.

The only FDA-approved medication for agitation in dementia is brexpiprazole, though it is no safer or better than other antipsychotics. Risperidone is approved for agitation in Australia and the UK and is also approved for aggression and psychotic symptoms for people with Alzheimer's dementia in Canada. Because these antipsychotics are only available in oral form and not as IVs or IMs, they are not appropriate for patients who require urgent treatment.

Treatment Recommendations

These recommendations are based in part on the following published algorithms: Chen A et al, *Psychiatry Research* 2021;295:113641; Davies SJC et al, *Journal of Psychopharmacology* 2018;32(5):509–523.

Constitutional measures

- Review any anticholinergic medications prescribed and reduce their dose or discontinue if feasible.
- Optimize bowel, pain, and sleep management
  - Bowel management: walking, prune juice, sennosides/docusate, bisacodyl, polyethylene glycol (MiraLAX), lactulose.
  - Pain:
    - Acetaminophen 325–650 mg q6h; used for agitation triggered by pain.
    - Morphine 2.5–10 mg q4h PRN; reserved for patients receiving hospice care.
  - Sleep: Melatonin 1–10 mg three hours before bedtime.

Antidementia therapies

If not already initiated, start treatment with an AChEI and/or memantine, as appropriate.

Antidepressants

- Antidepressants might seem like an unusual choice for the treatment of agitation in patients with dementia, but they have been helpful in studies and are frequently ordered.
- Antidepressants are not helpful in emergencies; instead, you will want to use intramuscular or intravenous options to achieve rapid control of dangerous behaviors.
- Antidepressants are a second-line choice for agitation in people with dementia after acetylcholinesterase inhibitors.
- Antidepressants, particularly selective serotonin reuptake inhibitors (SSRIs) and serotonin norepinephrine reuptake inhibitors (SNRIs), are preferred over antipsychotics in older adults. This is because they do not carry the same level of risk, including the black box warning for increased risk of death in patients with dementia. Additionally, antidepressants can be helpful in treating co-occurring depressive and anxiety symptoms, which can contribute to agitation and other behavioral disturbances.
- There is no significant difference in efficacy for agitation and psychotic symptoms between SSRIs and antipsychotics in people with dementia, so use them with confidence (Young JJ, *Am J Psychiat Res J* 2019;14(6):3-5).
- Specific medications
  - Positive results have been demonstrated with sertraline, trazodone, and citalopram for agitation. Paroxetine has had mixed outcomes, and trials with fluoxetine and fluvoxamine have failed (Young JJ 2019). Although prescribed frequently, there is a negative study for mirtazapine in treating agitation (Banerjee S et al, *Lancet* 2021;398(10310):1487–1497).
  - Escitalopram has been thought to be a safer alternative to citalopram but in a randomized controlled trial (RCT) was ineffective in treating agitation in AD and was associated with cardiac conduction delays and increased falls, suggesting that citalopram may be the preferred option (Rajji TK et al, *Nature Medicine* 2025 Mar 25:1-6).
  - The best overall evidence is for citalopram (Chen K et al, *Front Aging Neurosci* 2023;15:1103039). However, it is a second-line option in older adults due to a black box warning for QTc prolongation at higher doses. For most patients, use sertraline 25-200 mg daily as the first-line option.
  - For agitation in patients with frontotemporal dementia (FTD), trazodone 50–300 mg per day in divided doses is effective in reducing symptoms.
  - Dosing regimens and titration for antidepressants are similar to those used in the treatment of major depressive disorder.
  - It is important to note that antidepressants may require up to nine weeks to achieve full therapeutic effect, and patients may not experience any improvement during the first three weeks of treatment (Weintraub D et al, *Am J Geriatr Psychiatry* 2015;23(11):1127–1133). This delayed onset of action is crucial to convey to both patients and

caregivers. In inpatient settings and emergency departments, where rapid symptom control is often necessary, second-generation antipsychotics (SGAs) are frequently used to manage agitation.

Anticonvulsants

- Listed in order of preference
  - Gabapentin 300–900 mg daily in divided doses. Some patients may respond to higher doses. Watch for side effects, including dizziness. Renally dose in patients with kidney insufficiency.
  - Carbamazepine 50–400 mg daily in divided doses may help with hostility, aggression, or assaultive behavior. Monitor for side effects and drug-drug interactions, including decreased effect of donepezil. Therapeutic serum level may be around 5 micrograms/ml.
  - Divalproex/Valproic acid 125 mg qHS to 500 mg daily in divided doses. Due to limited efficacy and the risk of sedation, falls, hyponatremia, and neurotoxicity at moderate to higher doses, it is generally reserved for cases where other options have failed. It may offer more benefit in managing disinhibited behavior than outright aggression.

SGAs

- Black box warning
  - All antipsychotics carry a black box warning for increased risk of mortality in patients with dementia-related psychosis.
  - Estimated risk of death: ~2.3% with placebo versus ~3.5% with antipsychotics (a 1–2% absolute risk increase) (Schneider LS et al, *JAMA* 2005;294(15):1934-1943).
  - When discussing antipsychotics with caregivers, I will say something like: "I am concerned that [the patient] is in danger of harming themselves or others. For this reason, I am recommending an antipsychotic. One of these medications is FDA-approved for this indication. Unfortunately, all of these medications carry a small increase in the risk of death in patients with dementia. The risk is about 2.3% with sugar pills and 3.5% with these medications. So, there's a 1–2% higher chance of death. I wouldn't recommend [medication] unless I thought it was necessary. What are your thoughts?"
- Because of the black box warning, scheduled (standing) antipsychotics are reserved for the treatment of ongoing agitation in dementia where there is a risk of harm to the patient or others, significant distress that cannot be alleviated by nonpharmacological interventions, and a clinical need for symptom relief.
- FDA-approved options
  - Brexpiprazole
    - The only FDA-approved agent for agitation in Alzheimer's dementia.
    - Efficacy: Mild to moderate effect size of 0.31 (Lee D et al, *JAMA Neurol* 2023;80(12):1307-1316).
    - Safety: Similar risk to other SGAs, as it was associated with excess deaths in clinical trials compared to placebo.
- Recommended antipsychotics for agitation in dementia (listed in order of preference)
  - Aripiprazole: 2–15 mg daily
    - Moderate evidence for efficacy.
    - Relatively favorable side effect profile.
  - Risperidone: 0.25–2 mg daily
    - Approved for behavioral disturbances in dementia in several countries.
    - Effective for reducing aggression.
  - Olanzapine: 2.5–10 mg daily
    - Moderate efficacy for agitation but associated with significant metabolic side effects.
  - Brexpiprazole: 2–3 mg daily
    - Lower doses were ineffective in trials.
    - It is not recommended for PRN use
  - Quetiapine: 12.5–200 mg daily (divided doses)
    - A popular choice, including for patients with Parkinson's disease dementia (PDD) or dementia with Lewy bodies (DLB).
    - Less effective in studies compared to other SGAs.
- Special considerations for agitation in dementia subtypes
  - AD and Vascular Dementia (VaD):
    - Preferred medications: Aripiprazole, risperidone, olanzapine, and brexpiprazole.
  - DLB or PDD:
    - Avoid higher-potency antipsychotics, which will worsen motor symptoms and increase mortality.
    - Recommended: Low doses of quetiapine or clozapine.

- Duration of treatment
  - Behavioral symptoms in dementia are often transient.
  - Taper to the lowest effective dose or discontinue the antipsychotic once symptoms stabilize to reduce long-term risks.

Combinations

Antidepressants, anticonvulsants, and SGAs. Avoid combining SGAs.

Adrenaline-mediated treatments (limited data, though recommended in recent algorithms)

- Prazosin 1–6 mg daily in divided doses; watch for orthostatic hypotension.
- Propranolol 10–100 mg daily in divided doses; watch for bradycardia and hypotension (Peskind ER et al, *Alzheimer Dis Assoc Disord* 2005;19(1):23–28).

Electroconvulsive therapy (ECT)

- Trial ultra-brief right unilateral pulses over bilateral ECT initially.
- Risk of increased confusion.

Agitation in Dementia: Nonpharmacological Treatment

Nonpharmacological interventions are the first-line treatment of agitation in patients with dementia due to their better safety profile and effectiveness, though they are unsuitable in situations where immediate results are needed. Many patients will respond to a combination of specially tailored treatments. Music, simulated presence, validation therapy, and caregiver education have the strongest evidence for reducing agitation (Meyer C and O'Keefe, *Dementia* 2020;19(6):1927-1954).

Behavioral Interventions

Validation therapy

- *Description:* Avoid contradicting the patient. No one likes to be refuted or told "no," and the same holds for people with dementia, but since their coping mechanisms may be reduced, they may be more likely to act out when frustrated. Instead of confrontation, acknowledge and validate the patient's feelings and experiences.
- *Implementation*
  - Active listening: Listen attentively and empathically without correcting.
  - Validation phrases: Use statements like "I understand this is very upsetting for you."
  - Nonjudgmental: Avoid correcting or confronting the person's perceptions.
  - Tone of voice: Use a calm, gentle, and reassuring tone.
  - Body language: Use open and nonthreatening body language. Avoid crossing arms or standing over the person.
- *Examples*
  - Scenario 1: If a patient believes they need to go home to care for their children (who are now adults), instead of correcting them, say, "You must've been a wonderful parent to be so concerned about your kids."
  - Scenario 2: If a patient is anxious about an imagined event, respond with, "It sounds like that's really worrying you. Tell me more about it."

Redirecting attention

- *Description:* Distract the patient from something that is upsetting them with an alternative activity.
- *Implementation*
  - Activities: Introduce activities such as puzzles, music, or simple crafts.
  - Redirection techniques: Gently guide conversations or actions to a different topic or activity.
- *Examples*
  - Scenario 1: Losing items— Patient says, "Who took my glasses? I can't find them anywhere!" Respond with:
    - Validation: "It must be really upsetting not to find your glasses."
    - Redirection: "Let's take a break and have a snack. Maybe they'll turn up later."
  - Scenario 2: Resisting activities of daily living—Patient says, "I don't want to take a bath! Leave me alone!" Respond with:
    - Validation: "I understand that you don't want to take a bath right now."
    - Redirection: "How about we start by just washing your hands with some warm, soapy water? It'll feel really nice and refreshing."
  - Scenario 3: Disorientation to location—Patient says, "I need to go home now!" even though they are at home. Respond with:
    - Validation: "You must miss your home a lot."
    - Redirection: "Before we go, can you help me water the plants here? They always perk up when you take care of them."
  - Scenario 4: Repeating questions or statements—Patient keeps asking, "Where is Mom? I need to talk to her." Respond with:
    - Validation: "It sounds like you're really missing your mom today."
    - Redirection: "Let's look at some family photos. I have a beautiful album we can look at together."

Sensory Interventions

Music therapy

- *Description:* Play music to soothe and engage patients. Patients will respond best to music from their youth or to music played at memorable events like a wedding.
- *Implementation*
  - Personalized playlists: Curate music based on the patient's preferences and past experiences.
  - Live music: If possible, involve live music sessions or sing-alongs. They are received better than prerecorded music.

- *Questions for caregivers*
  - "What type of music does the patient enjoy?"
  - "Can music be integrated into the daily routine?"
- *Evidence:* Studies indicate that music therapy can reduce agitation, anxiety, and apathy, as well as promote well-being and sociability (Scales K et al, *The Gerontologist* 2018;58(s1):S88–S102).

Simulated presence therapy (SPT)

- *Description:* SPT uses pre-recorded messages from family members or close friends to replicate their presence, providing emotional support and comfort to individuals with dementia.
- *Implementation*
  - Create personalized recordings: Record messages from family or other loved ones that include familiar stories, expressions of love, or reassurances. The content should be short (5-10 minutes), positive, and comforting. Use audio or video recordings depending on what the individual responds to best.
  - Schedule: Play the recordings at times when the individual is most likely to be agitated or anxious, such as during care, in the evenings, or before bedtime.
- *Example*
  - Scenario: Missing a family member
    - Patient: "Where is my daughter? I need to see her."
    - SPT recording: "Hi Mom, it's me, [Daughter's Name]. I'm thinking of you and sending you all my love. I'll be visiting you very soon, but until then, remember that you're always in my heart."

Aromatherapy

- *Description:* Use scents to calm and relax patients.
- *Implementation*
  - Essential Oils: Use calming scents such as lavender or lemon balm.
  - Diffusers: Place diffusers in living spaces to distribute scents.
- *Questions for caregivers*
  - "Are there any allergies or sensitivities to consider?"
  - "Can aromatherapy be combined with other relaxation techniques?"
- *Evidence:* Aromatherapy has been shown to decrease agitation and improve overall well-being in patients with dementia.

Social Interventions

Social interaction and support

- *Description:* Enhance social engagement.
- *Implementation*
  - Family visits: Encourage regular visits from family and friends.
  - Group activities: Facilitate social activities like games, crafts, or shared meals. Structured group activities are offered in senior centers, adult day programs, and assisted living or skilled nursing facilities.
- *Questions for caregivers*
  - "How often does the patient interact with others?"
  - "Are there opportunities for the patient to engage in social activities?"

Family caregiver interventions

- *Description:* Family caregiver interventions focus on educating and supporting caregivers to manage behavioral symptoms, including agitation. These interventions also aim to provide a supportive network where caregivers can share experiences, gain insights, and learn strategies for day-to-day care.
- *Implementation*
  - Caregiver education
    - Educate caregivers about common behavioral symptoms in dementia, their causes, and effective management strategies.
    - Provide handouts and direct caregivers to informative websites like alz.org (provides Alzheimer's dementia resources and psychoeducation).
    - Refer caregivers to local or online support groups where they can connect with others facing similar challenges.
  - Problem-solving
    - Work with caregivers to identify specific triggers of the patient's agitation to mitigate them.
    - Common triggers:
      - Change in routine
      - Constipation

        - Disorientation
        - Fear
        - Hunger
        - Infections
        - Loss of control
        - Over/understimulation
        - Pain
        - Change in environment (eg, being hospitalized or leaving home for a few days)
    - Develop personalized strategies to address these triggers using nonpharmacological methods.
  - Task modifications
    - Reduce the complexity of the patient's environment and daily tasks to decrease potential stressors that could precipitate agitation.
    - Train caregivers in techniques to improve communication with the person with dementia, recognizing that clear, simple interactions can reduce frustrations for both the caregiver and the patient.
    - Encourage and facilitate the increase of suitable activities that match the patient's abilities and interests to promote engagement and reduce agitation.
- *Evidence*
  - The approach with the strongest evidence base in managing agitation in people with dementia is caregiver education and support. It has been shown to have a greater effect on agitation than antipsychotic medications (Kales HC et al, *BMJ* 2015;350:h369).

Apathy in Dementia: Diagnosis and Treatment

Apathy is the most common behavioral disturbance in dementia, impacting up to 36% of patients with dementia and 12%–40% of people with mild cognitive impairment (MCI) (Lyketsos CG et al, *JAMA* 2002 288(12):1475-1483). It is almost universally present in patients with severe dementia but may also be the first sign of dementia in some individuals. Associated with increased conversion from MCI to dementia and worsened disease progression, apathy has been linked with impaired everyday functioning, increased caregiver burden, worsened adherence to interventions, and worsened quality of life (Burgon C et al, Dement *Geriatr Cogn Disord* 2021;50(2):111–123).

Diagnosis

Definition

Apathy is characterized by a lack of interest, enthusiasm, or concern. In older adults, apathy may manifest as diminished motivation to perform daily activities, a lack of emotional response to situations that would typically elicit feelings, or a general sense of indifference.

Clinical interview tips

Ask the patient and their family about specific examples of changes in behavior, such as reduced participation in previously enjoyed hobbies or decreased social interactions. Explore how apathy affects the patient's daily functioning, including self-care, social relationships, and overall quality of life.

Differentiation from depression

- Both apathy and depression involve a loss of interest in activities and decreased motivation. This overlap can make it challenging to distinguish between the two.
- People who are depressed have symptoms like persistent sadness, feelings of worthlessness or excessive guilt, significant changes in sleep and appetite, and thoughts of death or suicide.
- People who are apathetic are indifferent or have a lack of emotional responsiveness rather than the emotional pain and suffering that accompany depression.
- It is important to distinguish between the two because they have different treatment strategies.

Scales

The Neuropsychiatric Inventory Questionnaire (NPI-Q) has one easy-to-remember question for apathy: Does the patient seem less interested in their usual activities or in the activities and plans of others? (Kaufer DI et al, J *Neuropsychiatry Clin Neurosci* 2000;12(2):233-239).

Treatment

Educate caregivers

- Apathy is one of the most common features of dementia.
- Use gentle commands to motivate instead of asking, as patients will often decline requests. For example, instead of asking, "Do you want lunch?" say, "It's time for lunch."
- Choose battles wisely. For example, if there is resistance to bathing, rather than insisting on daily baths, switch to every other day or try again later.
- Engage patients in stimulating activities like watching a favorite movie, listening to music, or looking at pictures of friends or family together.
- Consider enrolling patients in an adult day program or senior center for further engagement and daily structure.
- Emphasize the importance of a regular daily routines.

Medications

There are no FDA-approved treatments for apathy, see table for off-label options.

Table 34: **Medications for Apathy in Dementia**

Medication Class	Drug	Dosage	Considerations
Antidepressants	Bupropion XL	150–300 mg qAM	Monitor for insomnia, agitation, and potential weight changes
Cholinesterase inhibitors and NMDA receptor antagonists	Cholinesterase inhibitors (eg, donepezil, rivastigmine) and memantine	Indicated for dementia treatment; may indirectly affect apathy by improving cognitive function	Not specific for apathy; consider as part of standard dementia care
Dopaminergic agents	Amantadine	300–900 mg daily in divided doses	Some evidence from studies; monitor for side effects such as depression, edema, falls, hallucinations, livedo reticularis, and orthostatic hypotension
	Methylphenidate	Start at 5 mg twice daily (morning and noon), titrate to 10 mg twice daily after 2 weeks as appropriate	Has the best evidence for apathy; monitor for agitation, restlessness, irritability, QTc prolongation, and weight loss
	Pramipexole	Start at 0.125 mg three times daily, titrate up to a max of 4.5 mg/day	Useful for apathy in people with Parkinson's disease dementia; monitor for hallucinations, delusions, impulse control disorders, and dyskinesias
	Ropinirole	Start at 0.25 mg three times daily, titrate up to 3 mg/day	Similar considerations as pramipexole

Source: Mintzer J et al, JAMA Neurol 2021;78(11):1324–1332; van Reekum R et al, J *Neuropsychiatry Clin Neurosci* 2005;17(1):7-19.

Depression in Dementia: Diagnosis and Treatment

The incidence of depression is up to 30% in patients with Alzheimer's dementia (AD) and even higher in people with vascular dementia (VaD) and dementia with Lewy bodies (DLB). Depression occurs in over 40% of patients with Parkinson's disease dementia (PDD) (Kitching D, *Aust Prescr* 2015;38(6):209–211). This fact sheet will address the use of antidepressants in people with dementia for the treatment of depression.

Clinical Presentation

- Patients with dementia may not report classic symptoms of depression like worthlessness, guilt, thoughts of death or suicide, and sleep disruption—though these should still be assessed—because of limited self-expression, reduced self-awareness, or alternative symptoms.
- Alternate symptoms include diminished affect, increased irritability, loss of pleasure with social experiences or preferred activities, and decreased spontaneous communication.
- Always assess for psychosis because one-third of depressed patients with dementia will experience delusions.

Diagnosis

Experts have suggested requiring three out of nine SIGECAPS symptoms, with at least one symptom of depressed mood or anhedonia/loss of interest, instead of the classic five out of nine SIGECAPS symptoms, for the diagnosis of depression in dementia (Olin JT et al, *Am J Geriatr Psychiatry* 2002;10(2):125–128).

Nonpharmacological Interventions

Holistic approach

- Involve caregivers in adding more structure to the older adult's routine, (eg, attending a senior center or having lunch with long-time friends).
- Connect with the older adult's primary care doctor to address comorbid medical conditions.
- Work to minimize medication side effects, improve nutritional status, and ameliorate sleep disturbances, all of which can impact mood and behavior.

Psychosocial interventions

Incorporate a broad range of psychosocial interventions, such as:

- Behavioral activation
- Conversation
- Environmental modifications
- Increased daily structure
- Music therapy
- Physical activity
- Reminiscence therapy

These techniques are covered in the following fact sheets: "Behavioral Activation for Older Adults with Depression," [page 50] "Reminiscence Therapy: Utilizing Past Memories for Mental Health," [page 146] "Physical Activity and Nutrition in Older Adults," [page 166] and "Complementary and Alternative Therapies for Older Adults" [page 169].

Pharmacological Interventions

- Introduce medications as part of a comprehensive approach that includes psychosocial interventions, as medications alone have limited efficacy in treating depression in people with dementia, though their benefits will usually outweigh their risks (Enache D et al, *Curr Opin Psychiatr* 2011;24(6):461-472).
- First-line medication options are sertraline or escitalopram.
- Mirtazapine has not been effective for core depressive symptoms in studies, though it is used frequently nonetheless to improve co-occurring insomnia and loss of appetite.
- Be vigilant about potential side effects (eg, falls, gastrointestinal upset, hyponatremia with serotonergic antidepressants).
- Improved mood can be exhibited by increased interaction with others, more facial expressions like smiling, greater activity level, and decreased irritability.

Diagnosis and Treatment of Psychosis in Dementia

Symptoms of psychosis are common in people with dementia. Delusions occur in 30% of patients, and hallucinations in 16% (Lyketsos CG et al, *JAMA* 2002 288(12):1475-1483). However, psychotic symptoms manifest differently in this population, and there are complexities in choosing antipsychotics, given the potential for severe side effects.

Diagnosis of Psychosis in Dementia

Hallucinations

- Hallucinations in patients with dementia are usually visual, unlike other psychiatric disorders where hallucinations are mostly auditory.
- Common visual hallucinations are of deceased relatives and friends.
- In dementia with Lewy bodies (DLB), patients experience visual hallucinations that can be both detailed and vivid (eg, seeing animals, children, or familiar people).
  - Example: A patient with DLB might recount seeing miniature French soldiers in his room at night, which he finds nonthreatening and even entertaining.
- Perception of these hallucinations varies greatly among individuals—some may view them as harmless or even mundane, others might find them unsettling and distressing.
  - Example: A patient with DLB may need to stop driving due to distressing hallucinations of children lying in the road, leading to a fear of accidentally hitting them.

Delusions

- These are usually related to the memory loss process and, except for paranoia, are different from what patients with psychotic disorders typically experience.
- Patients with dementia may:
  - Develop a belief that their personal belongings have been stolen, frequently targeting partners, caregivers, or staff. This delusion is often rooted in short-term memory impairment, in which patients forget the location of items and mistakenly conclude that they have been taken (Mizrahi R et al, *Am J Geriatr Psychiatry* 2006;14(7):573-581).
  - Believe their current residence is not their home and express a desire to "go home" because they no longer recognize their surroundings. Alternatively, they might search for a home from their past, such as their childhood house.
  - Believe that deceased friends and relatives are alive.
  - Think that others, including their partner or children, are strangers due to impaired facial recognition. They may also misidentify familiar people (eg, thinking their daughter is their wife).
  - Have paranoid thoughts (eg, accuse their partner of infidelity or think that strangers are trying to harm them).

Table 35: **Common Delusions in Patients with Dementia**

Type of Delusion	Description
Delusions of Abandonment	A belief that friends or family members have abandoned them.
Misidentification Delusions	• **Capgras delusion:** Belief that an imposter has replaced a loved one. • **Fregoli delusion:** Idea that strangers are familiar people in disguise.
One's House is Not One's Home	The patient may feel that their home is not their actual home and express a desire to "go home."
Paranoid Delusions	• Patients may conclude that others are conspiring against them, stealing from them, or otherwise intending them harm. • **Theft delusion:** Belief that caregivers or family have stolen personal items. • **Infidelity delusion:** Thoughts that their partner is unfaithful with no evidence.
Phantom Boarder Delusion	The patient may believe that strangers or additional people reside in their home.
Reduplicative Paramnesia	The belief that a place or location has been duplicated, existing in two or more places simultaneously, or that it has been "relocated" to another site.
Time-Shifting Delusion	The patient might think that deceased relatives or friends are still alive and present.

Treatment

Caregiver recommendations

Caregiver education is the primary treatment for mild symptoms that produce little distress or do not cause the patient to be dangerous to self or others. I recommend caregivers:

- Avoid arguing with or confronting patients about hallucinations or delusions.

- Distract patients by changing topics or starting an activity (eg, folding clothes, listening to music, watching a movie together).
- Respond to the distress or emotion conveyed by the hallucinations or delusions instead of their content, such as acknowledging that the patient is missing family or friends who have passed away.

Antipsychotics

- Antipsychotics are used to treat psychosis in people with dementia when:
  - Symptoms cause significant distress to the patient.
  - There is a risk of harm to the patient or others.
  - Nonpharmacological approaches have failed, and symptom relief is essential.
- Black box warning
  - Antipsychotics should not be used as first-line treatments due to their risks in this population, including increased mortality and adverse effects. They should be prescribed only after a thorough evaluation of risks and benefits and with ongoing monitoring.
  - All antipsychotics carry a black box warning for causing increased mortality in people with dementia-related psychosis.
  - The risk of death is higher with antipsychotics (3.5%) compared to placebo (2.3%), with common causes of death including cardiovascular events and infections (Schneider LS et al, *JAMA* 2005;294(15):1934-1943).
- FDA-approved and off-label options
  - Pimavanserin (FDA-approved for Parkinson's disease psychosis)
    - Indications: First-line treatment for psychosis in people with Parkinson's disease.
    - Mechanism: Selective serotonin inverse agonist at 5-HT2A receptors.
    - Efficacy: Delayed onset of action compared to traditional antipsychotics but it has minimal impact on motor symptoms (Pagan FL et al, *CNS Drugs* 2024;38(5):333–347).
    - Dose: 34 mg daily.
    - Safety: May cause QTc prolongation. Monitor ECG in patients with cardiac risks.
  - Aripiprazole
    - Indications: Effective for psychosis in AD.
    - Dose: 2–15 mg daily.
    - Safety: Fewer metabolic side effects compared to olanzapine but may cause akathisia.
  - Olanzapine
    - Indications: Effective for psychosis in AD.
    - Dose: 2.5–10 mg daily.
    - Safety: Associated with metabolic side effects, including weight gain and hyperglycemia.
  - Quetiapine
    - Indications: Preferred for psychosis in people with Parkinson's disease or DLB due to lower risk of worsening motor symptoms.
    - Dose: 12.5–200 mg daily (divided doses).
    - Safety: Less effective compared to other antipsychotics but better tolerated in these populations.
  - Risperidone
    - Indications: Approved in several countries for psychosis in Alzheimer's dementia (AD).
    - Efficacy: Effective for psychotic symptoms in AD.
    - Dose: 0.25–2 mg daily.
    - Safety: Greater risk of extrapyramidal symptoms (EPS), sedation, and strokes at higher doses.
- Choosing the right medication
  - AD or vascular dementia (VaD):
    - Recommended agents (in order of preference): Risperidone, aripiprazole, olanzapine, quetiapine.
    - Brexpiprazole may be considered if agitation coexists with psychosis.
  - DLB or Parkinson's disease dementia (PDD):
    - First-line: Pimavanserin (minimal impact on motor function).
    - Second-line: Low-dose quetiapine or clozapine (preferred for avoiding motor side effects).
    - Avoid high-potency antipsychotics, such as risperidone or olanzapine, which exacerbate parkinsonism and increase mortality.

Addressing Wandering and Sundowning in Patients with Dementia

Wandering and sundowning are challenging behaviors observed in patients with dementia. Effective management requires a comprehensive approach combining nonpharmacological and pharmacological interventions.

Sundowning

CASE VIGNETTE: *Ms. Goldman, an 85-year-old woman with dementia with Lewy bodies (DLB), exhibits increased agitation and confusion in the evenings, starting consistently around 5 pm.*

Definition

Sundowning is the emergence of agitation, restlessness, and other neuropsychiatric symptoms (NPS) beginning in the late afternoon or early evening.

Epidemiology

More than 20% of patients with Alzheimer's disease (AD) and other dementias may experience sundowning. It is correlated with institutionalization, injuries, faster cognitive decline, and greater caregiver burden (Canevelli M et al, Front Med 2016;3:73).

Etiology

Sundowning has been associated with decreased light exposure and dysregulation of the body's natural sleep-wake cycles, leading to a delirium-like state (Boronat AC et al, J Am Med Dir Assoc 2019;20(6):664-671).

Diagnosis

Based on clinical observation and caregiver reports.

Nonpharmacological interventions

First-line choice for treatment, but more severe cases often require supplementation with early evening and bedtime medications.

Table 36: **Nonpharmacological Interventions for Sundowning**

Intervention	Description
Adequate Daytime Lighting	Ensure bright lighting during the afternoon or early evening hours. This can be done by exposure to sunlight or a light box at 1,000 to 3,000 lux.
Calm Evening Environment	Minimize unnecessary noises, such as commotion from visitors, loudspeakers, dish banging, and loud staff conversations (in facilities), which can happen during evening shift changes.
Consistent Sleep Routine	• Maintain a regular sleep-wake cycle to improve circadian rhythm. • Discourage afternoon napping. This can decrease the impetus to sleep at night. Patients can also wake up disoriented from naps, thinking that it's morning, or they can wake up feeling more energized.
Daytime Activity Engagement	Encourage physical and mental activities during the day to reduce evening restlessness. Time spent walking has been inversely correlated with sundowning behaviors.
Early Dinner	Serve dinner early in the evening to prevent hunger-related agitation later.
Limit Stimulants	Avoid caffeine and other stimulants in the afternoon and evening.

Source: Canevelli M et al, *Front Med* 2016.

Pharmacological interventions for sundowning

- There are no established algorithms for managing sundowning.
- Typically, a low dose of medication is given about an hour before the patient begins to experience sundowning, followed by a slightly larger dose at bedtime to help with sleep and to reestablish the circadian rhythm. Evening and nighttime medications should also be paired with exposure to bright light in the morning.

Neurocognitive Disorders

Table 37: **Pharmacological Interventions for Sundowning**

Medication	Initial Dose	Side Effects	Timing
Melatonin	1–3 mg	Dizziness, headache	Administer 1 mg at 4 pm, then 3 mg at 7 pm, dose can be increased if needed
Trazodone	25 mg	Falls, hypotension, orthostatic, sedation	Administer 25 mg at 5 pm and 25–50 mg at HS, adjust based on response
Mirtazapine	7.5 mg	Sedation, weight gain	Administer at bedtime and adjust based on response
Quetiapine	12.5 mg	Metabolic syndrome, orthostatic hypotension, sedation	Administer 12.5–25 mg at 4 pm, then 25–50 mg at HS, adjust based on response
Olanzapine	1.25 mg	Anticholinergic symptoms, metabolic syndrome	Administer 1.25 mg at 4 pm and 1.25–2.5 mg at HS, adjust based on response

---

CASE CONT'D: *You decide to start melatonin 1 mg at 4 pm and 3 mg after dinner. Family reports that Ms. Goldman's agitation improves with melatonin but that the patient continues to have difficulty falling asleep at night. You add 25 mg of trazodone at bedtime with good results.*

Wandering

Definition

Aimless or confused movement, sometimes leading to dangerous situations.

Consequences

Wandering significantly increases the possibility of falls, injuries, and fractures. Patients who wander are at risk of becoming lost or missing from their homes or facilities. In some tragic instances, patients may inadvertently walk on to busy roads and suffer severe injuries or fatalities from motor vehicle accidents.

Risk factors

- People with AD and DLB are more likely to wander. Visuospatial dysfunction is a hallmark of AD and DLB, making it more probable for people with these forms of dementia to get lost in familiar places or have difficulty finding their way home from unfamiliar locales.
- Wandering has been linked to severe cognitive impairment (ie, a Mini-Mental State Examination (MMSE) score of 12 or less), in people with preserved ambulation (Agrawal AK et al, *Indian J Psychol Med* 2021;43(5S):53S–59S).

Evaluation

Investigate whether there are modifiable triggers present, including boredom from lack of stimulation; overall restlessness; increased disorientation in the evening and night; physical symptoms such as hunger or pain not being addressed; akathisia from antipsychotic medications or undiagnosed restless legs syndrome; or psychosis (eg, paranoia may cause the person to try to escape from what they perceive as a dangerous situation).

Nonpharmacological strategies

Should be the first-line approach due to their safety and efficacy

- Traditional management is comprised of physical barriers and monitoring devices.
- A new attitude toward the management of wandering has evolved, with a move toward promoting safe walking areas rather than preventing wandering.
- GPS trackers and similar interventions raise ethical issues because they could be unwanted or coercive (Cipriani G et al, *Psychogeriatrics* 2014;14:135-142).
- The ultimate decision regarding whether to implement an intervention for wandering should include a balance of considering the need for patient safety, informed consent, and ethical principles like autonomy.

Table 38: **Nonpharmacological Interventions for Wandering**

Intervention	Description
Activities	Engage patients in meaningful activities that distract them from the urge to wander.
Alerting Local Police	Inform local authorities about the patient's condition so they can respond quickly if the patient is found wandering.
Cameras and GPS Trackers	• Cameras and GPS trackers monitor patients' movements and help to quickly locate them if they leave a safe environment. • GPS devices are manifold and include watches, wristbands, personal locators, tags, and even shoe soles.
Change the Locks on Doors	Use locks that are difficult for the patient to operate, such as those higher up, or those disguised as something else.
Companionship and Supervision	Increase supervision and provide companionship during times when the person is most likely to wander. This might involve having family stay with them overnight or hiring in-home help, such as a home health aide.
Environmental Modifications	• Secure the environment with locked doors, alarms, or barriers. • Use visual cues, such as STOP signs on doors, to redirect patients. • Wander guards for homes and facilities prevent doors from opening if the person attempts to exit the premises. • Bed alarms activate when an individual gets out of bed. They can alert caregivers at night that the patient is up and about.
Exercise Programs	Plan regular physical activity during the day, including walking, tailored to the patient's ability, to reduce restlessness and improve sleep patterns.
Medical ID Bracelets	Ensure patients wear medical ID bracelets with important information, such as diagnosis, caregiver contact, and urgent medical needs.
Safe Walking Paths	Designate safe areas for walking within the home or facility to allow movement without risk.
Structured Daily Routines	Establish a predictable routine to provide a sense of stability and reduce confusion.
Wander Bracelet or Necklace	Equip patients with a wander bracelet or necklace to help identify them and alert caregivers if they wander.

Pharmacological interventions for wandering

- There are no published drug strategies to manage wandering.
- Medications can be considered in cases where a patient's safety is threatened, such as for someone wandering at night onto major thoroughfares or getting lost.
- Utilize the algorithm for nonurgent treatment of behavioral agitation in people with dementia, with an emphasis on anti-dementia drugs, selective serotonin reuptake inhibitors/selective serotonin norepinephrine reuptake inhibitors, and second-generation antipsychotics.
- If wandering occurs mainly at night, focus on improving sleep by employing medications; see "Table 37: Pharmacological Interventions for Sundowning."

Inappropriate Sexual Behaviors in Dementia

Dementia is usually accompanied by apathy and decreased sexual interest, but disinhibition and inappropriate sexual behaviors (ISBs) can emerge in up to 18% of community-dwelling older adults with dementia. They are most commonly linked to male sex and anxiety. These behaviors can be troublesome for caregivers and disruptive in shared settings like nursing homes (Canevelli et al, *Am J Geriatr Psychiatry* 2017;25(4):365-371).

Types

- *Verbal behaviors:* Explicit or socially inappropriate sexual remarks or requests.
- *Sexual acts:* Touching, grabbing, or exposing genitals or public masturbation.
- *Implied behaviors:* Openly viewing pornographic material or requesting unnecessary genital care.

Diagnosis

(Proposed criteria adapted from: Sachdev P, *Am J Geriatr Psychiatry* 2017;25(4):372-373)

- The individual is diagnosed with dementia and engages in sexual behavior, verbal or physical, that is new in onset since diagnosis.
- The behavior is considered inappropriate for any of the following reasons
  - It is carried out in a public place and is offensive to others.
  - It is directed at persons who find it unacceptable.
  - It is directed toward persons unwilling or unable to consent.
  - It is excessive and interferes with daily activities.
  - It poses a risk of harm to the individual or others.
  - The individual shows an inability to control the behavior.

Causes

- *Frontal lobe dysfunction*, such as in frontotemporal dementia (FTD), may impair social awareness and the ability to inhibit urges.
- *Medical/psychiatric comorbidities:* Conditions like Parkinson's disease (PD), strokes, head injuries, delirium, and bipolar mania can result in sexual disinhibition.
- *Medication side effects:* Medications, including dopaminergics for PD and benzodiazepines for anxiety and insomnia, can trigger disinhibited behavior and hypersexuality.
- *Social factors:* There are often constraints in long-term care settings that might impede private sexual activity leading to a public display. Bathing or hygiene care provided by staff may also be misinterpreted as a sexual act or romantic advance by some patients (Srinivasan S and Weinberg AD, *Annals of Long-Term Care* 2006;14(10):20-28).

Assessment

Take a thorough history, including a sexual history. Determine whether the behavior is truly "inappropriate" or a value judgment. Screen for medical illness, including delirium, and cognitive impairment.

Management Strategies

Nonpharmacological

- Distraction techniques include social activity (snacks, drinks, conversations, exercising, and walking) and involvement in crafts that occupy the hands, thereby preventing touching or masturbation.
- Address unmet needs like loneliness or boredom.
- Environment changes such as switching staff members, avoiding overstimulating television programs or magazines, moving to a single room, providing opportunities for healthy and safe sexual expression, and clothing modifications may all help.
- Provide education to caregivers, staff, and family members about late-life sexuality, ISBs, and strategies for managing challenging behaviors.

Pharmacological

No randomized controlled trials for ISB exist. Medications are used after nonpharmacological strategies have failed. Anti-androgens can be highly effective in complex cases but pose ethical concerns. Table 39 lists medication options in order of suggested trials.

Table 39: **Medications to Treat Inappropriate Sexual Behaviors in Dementia**

Medication Class	Medications and Daily Doses
Antidepressants	Escitalopram 10–20 mg Mirtazapine 15–30 mg Trazodone 100–500 mg
Mood stabilizers	Carbamazepine 200–800 mg Gabapentin 300–900 mg
Antipsychotics	Haloperidol 1.5–3 mg Quetiapine 25–75 mg
Cholinesterase inhibitors	Rivastigmine 3–12 mg
Beta and histamine blockers	Cimetidine 400–1600 mg Pindolol 10–40 mg Propranolol 80–160 mg
Hormonal agents	Cyproterone acetate 10 mg Medroxyprogesterone 200–500 mg IM

Source: De Giorgi R and Series H, *Curr Treat Options Neurol* 2016;18(9):41; Sarangi A et al, *Cureus* 2021;13(10):e18463; Srinivasan S et al, *Curr Psychiatry Rep* 2019;21(10):97.

Reminiscence Therapy: Utilizing Past Memories for Mental Health

In reminiscence therapy (RT), patients recall positive experiences and memories from the past. It is a useful treatment for older adults with memory loss or depression and can help foster a sense of well-being. While RT is usually done in group settings, this fact sheet will introduce some key features that can be incorporated into brief office visits and taught to caregivers for home use.

Why Do Reminiscence Therapy?

- *Boosts cognition:* RT stimulates long-term memories, providing cognitive benefits for individuals with neurocognitive disorders.
- *Depression in older adults:* RT has been shown to promote life satisfaction and alleviate depression in meta-analyses (Xu L et al, *Front Psychiatry* 2023;14:1139700).
- *Builds connections:* When delivered via group sessions, RT encourages sharing and bonding, thereby reducing loneliness and fostering a supportive social network.
- *Strengthens identity:* Reflecting on past achievements and life events helps maintain a sense of personal identity and continuity over time.
- *Encourages closure:* RT offers a chance to think about life's journey, resolve old issues, and impart wisdom, contributing to personal fulfillment.

When to Use Reminiscence Therapy?

- *Early stages of dementia:* Can be helpful in the early stages of Alzheimer's dementia (AD) to improve cognition, depression, activities of daily living, and quality of life. Patients with mild to moderate AD respond best to photographs, videos, and music linked with personal past experiences (Cuevas PEG et al, *Int J Ment Health Nurs* 2020;29(3):364-371). RT is less effective in late-stage dementia.
- *End-of-life care:* In hospice care settings, RT can provide comfort, facilitate life review, and help individuals find meaning and peace in their final days.

Essential Tools

These tools can be used during appointments or taught to caregivers for use at home.

- *Memory boxes:* Ask caregivers to create a personal memory box for the patient, filled with small, meaningful items from their past (eg, photographs, letters, mementos, other objects). During a short session, one item from the box can be selected for discussion while the patient is guided through the memories it evokes.
- *Themed conversation cards:* Develop a set of cards, each representing a different life theme (eg, family, holidays, hobbies). In a brief session, the patient can choose a card and share memories related to the theme. This can spur spontaneous conversation and reminiscence.
- *Playlists:* Music can be a powerful trigger for memory recall. A short session might involve listening to a song or two from the past and discussing the memories brought up.
- *Photo albums:* Encourage caregivers to organize photo albums with labels and short descriptions. Flipping through a few photos can trigger memories and discussions.
- *Story prompts:* Prepare a list of story prompts or questions tailored to the patient's life history (eg, "Tell me about your first job" or "What was your wedding day like?")

Training Caregivers

- *Empathy and patience:* Emphasize the importance of showing empathy and patience. Encourage caregivers to listen attentively and validate the patient's feelings and memories, as well as to focus on positive memories, while avoiding arguments or contradicting the patient.
- *Guidance on tool use:* Provide clear instructions on how to use each tool and technique. For example, demonstrate how to select a photo from an album and use open-ended questions to encourage the patient to share memories.

Sample Questions to Provoke Reminiscence

- *Initiating the session*
  - "Today, let's take a trip down memory lane. Is there a particular time in your life you'd like to start with?"
  - "I noticed this photo/music/object catches your interest. Can you tell me more about it?"
- *Encouraging detailed recollections*
  - "That sounds like a special moment. Can you describe what that day was like?"
  - "How did you feel when that happened? What do you remember most vividly?"
  - "Who was with you at that time, and what was your relationship with them like?"
- *Validating emotions and experiences*
  - "It sounds like that was a really important time for you."

- "I imagine that must have been challenging/exciting for you. How did you manage?"
- *Navigating difficult memories*
  - "If this memory is painful and you'd rather not talk about it right now, that's okay. We can discuss something else or take a break."
  - "It's brave of you to share that with me. Would you like to explore how that experience has shaped you, or would you prefer to shift to another memory?"
- *Connecting past to present*
  - "How do you think those experiences have influenced you today?"
  - "What did you learn from that time in your life?"
- *Closing the reverie*
  - "Thank you for sharing these memories today. Is there anything else you'd like to add or a different memory you'd like to discuss in the future?"
  - "I've enjoyed hearing about your life and the experiences that have meant so much to you."
- *Providing support and encouragement*
  - "You've lived through some remarkable times, and your stories are incredibly valuable."
  - "It's been an honor to listen to your stories. You have a rich history that deserves to be celebrated."

Clinical Scenarios and Responses

CASE VIGNETTE 1: *Mr. Ahmad, a retired veteran, often feels disconnected from his family, who, he says, does not understand his past. Using a memory box, his caregiver brings out medals and photos from his service time, asking about the stories behind each item. This stimulates Mr. Ahmad's memory and provides a tangible way for his family to connect with his experiences.*

CASE VIGNETTE 2: *Mrs. Brooks, an individual in the early stages of dementia, struggles with short-term memory loss. Her caregiver utilizes old photographs. By presenting visual cues, such as pictures of flowers Mrs. Brooks once grew, the caregiver is able to initiate conversations that resonate with Mrs. Brooks's interests. This approach not only stimulates cognitive function but also brings joy and a sense of identity to Mrs. Brooks*

CASE VIGNETTE 3: *Mr. Hoffman, who is usually withdrawn, has a deep love for classical music. A short visit involves playing a piece of music from his collection. This leads Mr. Hoffman to vividly recount seeing the performance live, showcasing how music can bridge communication gaps and stimulate memory.*

Resources

Books

Reminiscence and Life Story Work: A Practice Guide, Fourth Edition by Faith Gibson focuses on using life stories and reminiscence in care settings, providing a practical approach to implementing these techniques.

Online resources and websites

Caregivers Activity Source (https://tinyurl.com/3f8ssde7): Contains activities to stimulate reminiscence that can be used with older adults.

Manuals

- Age UK (https://tinyurl.com/yt9fvfdb): Offers a free manual on reminiscence and life story work, that includes information on activities that stimulate recollecting and therapy.
- The Benevolent Society (https://tinyurl.com/3cvywwft): Has a free and short Reminiscing Handbook, which contains many practical tips for helping people reminisce, including having successful conversations and creating memory kits.

Medication Management and Neuromodulation

Basics of Psychopharmacology in Older Adults

Psychopharmacology in older adults is uniquely complicated by age-related changes in drug metabolism, increased sensitivity to side effects, and the frequent presence of comorbid medical conditions. Polypharmacy is common, necessitating careful consideration of drug-drug interactions and overall medication burden. As a result, clinicians should follow the principle of "start low and go slow" to balance efficacy with safety.

Cytochrome P450 System

Aging leads to slowed metabolism via the CYP450 system. This significantly impacts the CYP1A2 and CYP3A enzymes but not CYP2D6, which has more resilience to the aging process.

- *Implication:* Potential for elevated blood levels of psychotropic drugs metabolized by the CYPA enzymes. Impacted agents include:
  - Antipsychotics (aripiprazole, clozapine, lurasidone, quetiapine, and ziprasidone)
  - Benzodiazepines (excluding lorazepam, oxazepam, temazepam)
  - Others: carbamazepine, buspirone, methadone, and trazodone
- *Recommendation:* Either avoid substrates of CYP1A2 and CYP3A3/4 or prescribe smaller doses of medications metabolized by them and increase doses more slowly.

Fat Solubility and Accumulation

There are increased fat stores in later life. Most psychotropics are fat-soluble.

- *Implication:* Psychotropics will be absorbed extensively into fat cells, where they will be stored, leading to slow release, and with time, increased risk of drug toxicity. Some of the most prominently impacted medications are:
  - *Benzodiazepines*
  - *Clozapine*
  - *Fluoxetine*
  - *Haloperidol*
  - *Olanzapine*
- *Recommendation*: Prescribe smaller doses more frequently rather than larger doses less frequently.

Water-Soluble Drugs and Kidney Function

Aging results in decreased body water and reduced kidney clearance of drugs.

- *Implications:* Water-soluble medications will have higher circulating concentrations, increasing the risk of drug toxicity. Impacted agents include:
  - Lithium
  - Desvenlafaxine
  - Gabapentin
  - Paliperidone
  - Pregabalin
- *Recommendation:* Increase doses of water-soluble medications slowly, target smaller doses, and lengthen dosing intervals. For lithium, target doses for older adults are 30% lower than for younger adults.

Other Important Tips for Prescribing in Older Adults

Anticholinergics

- Agents with anticholinergic properties increase the risk of cardiovascular compromise, cognitive impairment, constipation, falls and fractures, urinary retention which can contribute to urinary tract infections, and visual impairment from pupillary dilatation.
- When possible, avoid medications with strong anticholinergic properties in older adults, including:
  - Amitriptyline
  - Chlorpromazine
  - Benztropine
  - Clomipramine
  - Clozapine
  - Cyclobenzaprine
  - Desipramine
  - Diphenhydramine
  - Doxepin (>6 mg/day)
  - Hydroxyzine

– Nortriptyline
– Olanzapine
– Oxybutynin
– Paroxetine
– Perphenazine

(Source: AGS Beers Criteria®, J Am Geriatr Soc 2023;71(7):2052-2081)

Antidepressants

- *Bleeding:* Selective serotonin reuptake inhibitors (SSRIs) and serotonin-norepinephrine reuptake inhibitor (SNRIs) increase the risk of upper GI bleeding in older adults due to their inhibition of platelet serotonin uptake, which impairs platelet aggregation. This effect is particularly concerning in patients with a history of gastrointestinal (GI) bleeding, those taking anticoagulants (eg, warfarin), antiplatelet agents (eg, aspirin, clopidogrel), or NSAIDs. The risk is dose-dependent and highest with fluoxetine.
- *Falls:* Psychotropics increase the risk of falls. The odds of falling are highest with the following classes of meds (in order): 1) SSRIs, 2) long-acting benzodiazepines, 3) antidepressants, and 4) antipsychotics (Source: Seppala LJ et al, *J Am Med Dir Assoc* 2018;19(4):371.e11-371.e17). Use of these classes of medications in a patient with recurrent falls may need to be balanced against the risk for future falls.
- *Hyponatremia:* Increased probability with SSRIs/SNRIs, carbamazepine, and oxcarbazepine.

Antipsychotics

- *Black box warning:* Boxed warning for increased risk of stroke and death in dementia.
- *Cardiovascular:* Most antipsychotics increase the risk for QTc prolongation which can lead to torsades de Pointes (TdP) and sudden cardiac death.
- *Orthostatic hypotension:* Can contribute to falls and ischemic strokes. The risk is higher with certain drugs.
- *Parkinson's disease (PD):* Antipsychotics may counteract levodopa/dopamine agonist effects, contributing to bradykinesia. Exceptions include drugs with low or no dopamine D2 receptor binding activity. These agents are used preferentially to treat psychosis in patients with PD. They include:
  – Clozapine
  – Lumateperone
  – Pimavanserin (only agent FDA-approved for this indication)
  – Quetiapine
- *Tardive dyskinesia:* Doubled risk in older adults; clozapine has a lower risk, and others are debatable.

General Recommendations

- Due to slowed drug metabolism and elimination with aging, start low and go slow when starting and titrating medications, but keep going as many older adults will respond to the same final doses as younger adults.
- For most medications, start at one-half the usual dose and increase to the minimal effective dose after one to two weeks.
- Avoid making more than one medication change at a time.
- Minimize and simplify drug regimens when possible.
- Optimize existing medications before adding others.
- Be cautious with agents that are anticholinergic or can cause cardiac arrhythmias, confusion, daytime sedation, or orthostatic hypotension.

Managing Medication Side Effects in Older Adults

Older adults are particularly vulnerable to adverse drug reactions due to polypharmacy, medical comorbidities, and age-related changes in drug metabolism. This fact sheet will provide detailed information on common side effects and drug interactions in older adults, along with recommendations for management.

Managing Medication Side Effects

Anticholinergic side effects

> **CASE VIGNETTE 1:** *Ms. Thompson, a 63-year-old woman, is prescribed amitriptyline (Elavil) 25 mg qHS for insomnia and cyclobenzaprine 10 mg two times daily (BID) for muscle spasms in her legs. She presents with complaints of increased forgetfulness and blurry vision.*

- *The problem:* Anticholinergic medications can result in cognitive impairment, dry mouth, constipation, urinary retention, and blurred vision.
- *Management*
  - Avoid anticholinergics in older adults, when possible.
  - Use alternatives with lower anticholinergic burden, such as selective serotonin reuptake inhibitors (SSRIs) for depression (eg, escitalopram 10-20 mg daily); melatonin 1-3 mg nightly or trazodone 25-50 mg nightly for insomnia; or buspirone 10-30 mg daily in divided doses for anxiety.
  - For dry mouth
    - Hydration: Encourage frequent sips of water and sugar-free chewing gum or lozenges. Use a humidifier at night.
    - Saliva substitutes: Use artificial saliva substitutes, like Biotene or Oasis, if necessary.
  - For constipation
    - Dietary fiber: Increase dietary fiber intake with fruits, vegetables, and whole grains.
    - Hydration: Ensure adequate fluid intake.
    - Physical activity: Encourage regular physical activity to promote bowel movements.
    - Stool softeners: Use stool softeners like Docusate (Colace) 100 mg twice daily or bowel stimulants such as Senna 1-2 tabs qHS, if needed. Prune juice is an osmotic laxative that also contains fiber.
  - For urinary retention: Implement bladder training exercises, such as scheduled toileting breaks. Scheduled voiding every two to three hours can help to prevent bladder overdistention.

Bleeding risk

> **CASE VIGNETTE 2:** *Mr. Patel, a 71-year-old man, takes sertraline 100 mg daily for major depressive disorder and has started taking over-the-counter ibuprofen 400 mg every six hours for low back pain. He has a prior history of a gastrointestinal (GI) hemorrhage for which he was hospitalized.*

- *The problem:* Increased risk of GI bleeding when serotonergic antidepressants are combined with anticoagulant or antiplatelet agents. Higher-risk patients are those who are taking multiple anticoagulants or who have a history of GI hemorrhages.
- *Management*
  - Monitor for signs of bleeding, such as easy bruising, nosebleeds, dark stools, or hematuria.
  - Avoid or limit NSAIDs and aspirin. Consider acetaminophen for pain relief.
  - Cautious use of anticoagulants: Recommend newer anticoagulants with lower bleeding risk, if suitable and approved by other physicians.
    - For patients with moderate risk of GI bleeding, H2 antagonists may be sufficient and preferred due to their better side effect profile.
  - Consider gastroprotection in higher-risk patients
    - Protein-pump inhibitors should be the first choice due to their superior efficacy in preventing bleeding.
  - Consider antidepressants with lower bleeding risk, such as mirtazapine 7.5-30 mg nightly or bupropion XL 150-300 mg daily.

Hyponatremia

CASE VIGNETTE 3: *Ms. Khan, a 91-year-old, starts sertraline 50 mg daily for treatment of a major depressive episode. One week later, her sodium level is 128, down from her baseline of 137.*

- *The problem:* Serotonergic antidepressants can increase the release of antidiuretic hormone, leading to water retention and dilutional hyponatremia.
- *Symptoms*
  - Mild to moderate hyponatremia: Nausea, headache, confusion, fatigue, weakness, muscle cramps, or spasms.
  - Severe hyponatremia: Delirium, seizures, or coma.
- *Assessment*
  - Baseline serum sodium: Measure serum sodium levels before starting an SSRI/serotonin-norepinephrine reuptake inhibitor (SNRI) in older adults.
  - Regular monitoring: Check sodium levels one to two weeks after initiating therapy, following dose adjustments, and periodically during long-term use.
  - Thresholds
    - Mild hyponatremia: Serum sodium level 130-134 mmol/L
    - Moderate hyponatremia: Serum sodium level of 125-129 mmol/L
    - Severe hyponatremia: Serum sodium level less than 125 mmol/L
- *Management*
  - Mild hyponatremia: Refer to primary care provider for workup and treatment.
  - Moderate to severe hyponatremia: Recommend medical admission for slow sodium correction and symptomatic monitoring. Rapid sodium correction can result in permanent paralysis.
  - When to discontinue or reduce the dose of an antidepressant
    - Not all older adults with low sodium have syndrome of inappropriate antidiuretic hormone secretion (SIADH). In these cases, antidepressant therapy should be continued lest the patient suffer a recurrence of depression.
    - Once SIADH has been confirmed, and it is established that it is due to an SSRI/SNRI, consider either discontinuing the medication in cases of moderate to severe hyponatremia or reducing the dose in mild hyponatremia, with continued monitoring.
    - SIADH is confirmed by:
      - Low serum osmolality (<275 mOsm/kg) which arises as retained water dilutes the blood.
      - Elevated urine osmolality (>100 mOsm/kg) results from the urine becoming abnormally concentrated due to insufficient water excretion from the body.
      - Elevated urine sodium (>20 mmol/L) occurs as the kidneys excrete sodium to reduce excess body water. Normally, water would follow sodium, but this does not happen in cases of SIADH.

Metabolic syndrome

CASE VIGNETTE 4: *Mr. Bennett is a 67-year-old male with schizoaffective disorder. He is prescribed olanzapine 10 mg qHS and divalproex ER 750 mg qHS. He presents to the clinic for routine follow-up. His primary complaints include fatigue and recent weight gain of 12 pounds over the past six months, despite no significant changes to his diet or physical activity. His BMI is measured at 31.9 kg/m^2 and waist circumference at 42 inches.*

- *The problem:* Certain antipsychotics can result in weight gain, hyperglycemia, dyslipidemia, and hypertension.
- *Management*
  - Baseline and regular weight, fasting glucose, and lipid profile monitoring.
  - Encourage lifestyle modifications, including a balanced diet of fruits, vegetables, whole grains, lean proteins, and healthy fats. Urge at least 150 minutes of moderate-intensity aerobic exercise per week, eg, brisk walking.
  - Consider switching to lower-risk antipsychotics such as aripiprazole, brexpiprazole, cariprazine, or lurasidone if significant metabolic changes occur.
  - Metformin has been successfully used in younger populations for metabolic syndrome. In older adults, its use can be limited by impaired renal function, GI side effects, and B12 deficiency from long-term administration.

QTc prolongation

CASE VIGNETTE 5: *Ms. Turner is a 76-year-old woman admitted for a urinary tract infection. She is prescribed ciprofloxacin. She develops delirium and receives quetiapine for agitation. ECG reveals a QTc interval of 514 ms.*

- *The problem:* Older adults are at higher risk for QTc prolongation, which increases the risk of torsades de pointes and sudden cardiac death.
- *Management*
  - Baseline and periodic ECG monitoring.
  - Monitor and correct abnormal electrolytes (potassium, magnesium, calcium).
  - Recommend magnesium be kept greater than two.
  - Avoid combining antipsychotics with other QTc-prolonging drugs (eg, ciprofloxacin, methadone).
  - Use the lowest effective antipsychotic dose to minimize risk.
  - Consider discontinuing the antipsychotic if QTc interval exceeds 500 ms or if there is a 60 ms increase from baseline, unless cleared by cardiology.
  - The antipsychotic with the least impact on QTc intervals is aripiprazole. Others with less impact include brexpiprazole, cariprazine, and lurasidone.

Serotonin syndrome

CASE VIGNETTE 6: *Mr. Watanabe is a 68-year-old male. He takes venlafaxine 150 mg daily for depression and buspirone 10 mg TID for GAD. He hurts his knees playing pickleball and is prescribed tramadol. Within hours of the first dose, he develops shivering, sweating, and mild disorientation.*

- *The problem:* Serotonin syndrome results from excess serotonin. It is iatrogenic (brought on by drug interactions). Clinical features include:
  - Mental status changes: Agitation, confusion, hypomania.
  - Autonomic instability: Hyperthermia, diaphoresis, tachycardia, hypertension, dilated pupils.
  - Neuromuscular abnormalities: Tremor and rigidity. Hyperreflexia and myoclonus are hallmark features.

Table 40: **Common Drug-Drug Combinations Leading to Serotonin Syndrome**

Drug Class	Examples	Mechanism
SSRIs	Sertraline, Fluoxetine, Escitalopram	Increased serotonin levels
SNRIs	Venlafaxine, Duloxetine	Increased serotonin levels
MAOIs	Phenelzine, Tranylcypromine	Inhibited breakdown of serotonin
Tricyclics	Clomipramine	Increased serotonin levels
Opioids	Tramadol, Meperidine, Fentanyl	Serotonin reuptake inhibition
Antimigraine Agents	Sumatriptan, Rizatriptan	Serotonin agonism
Herbal Supplements	St. John's Wort	Increased serotonin levels
Antibiotics	Linezolid	MAOI properties
Anti-Nausea Agents	Ondansetron (Zofran), Metoclopramide	Serotonin receptor antagonism/ agonism
Cough Suppressants	Dextromethorphan	Serotonin reuptake inhibition
Lithium	Lithium carbonate	Increased serotonin release

- *Management*
  - Immediate actions
    - Discontinue all serotonergic agents.
    - Because serotonin syndrome is life-threatening, moderate and severe cases should be treated on a medical unit.

- Supportive care
  - Hydration: Ensure adequate IV hydration.
  - Cooling measures: For hyperthermia, use external chilling methods like cooling blankets and fans.
  - Monitoring: Continuous monitoring of vital signs, labs, and neurological status, preferably in an ICU setting for severe cases.
- Psychotropic medications (which may help)
  - Benzodiazepines, eg, lorazepam 2-4 mg or diazepam 5-10 mg, can control myoclonus and agitation.
  - Cyproheptadine is a serotonin receptor antagonist that directly counteracts excess serotonin's effects. Initial dose is 12 mg, followed by 2 mg every two hours until symptoms improve. Maximum dose is 32 mg/day.

Tardive dyskinesia (TD)

CASE VIGNETTE 7: *Ms. Carter, an 83-year-old woman with moderate dementia, has been taking risperidone 4 mg qHS for sundowning agitation. Her caregiver notes she has developed mild lip puckering.*

- *The problem*
  - TD is due to long-term antipsychotic exposure. Rates of TD are much higher in older adults. Even with second-generation antipsychotics, it has a prevalence of up to 21% (Carbon M et al, *J Clin Psychiatry* 2017;78(3):e264-e278).
- *Symptoms:* Involuntary, repetitive movements most often involving the lips, mouth, and hands but that can involve any muscle group.
- *Management*
  - Screen patients every six months for TD using the Abnormal Involuntary Movement Scale (AIMS) examination.
  - Taper off anticholinergic medications as they can worsen TD.
  - If possible, gradually taper off the antipsychotic medication.
  - If the patient is receiving a first-generation antipsychotic, consider switching to a second-generation antipsychotic.
  - If the patient is receiving a second-generation antipsychotic, consider switching to one with lower risk of TD, such as quetiapine or clozapine.
  - VMAT2 Inhibitors
    - If TD persists despite any of the above or if they are not viable options, then consider adding valbenazine (Ingrezza) 40-80 mg daily or deutetrabenazine (Austedo) 24-36 mg/day in divided doses.
    - Valbenazine is the preferred choice due to once daily administration.
    - Valbenazine interacts with CYP2D6 and CYP3A4 modulators, whereas deutetrabenazine interacts primarily with CYP2D6 modulators and is contraindicated in hepatic impairment.
    - Both are well tolerated, though monitor for depression and rare suicidality. Both can prolong QTc intervals.

Important Drug-Drug Interactions in Older Adults

Drug-drug interactions are critical to monitor in older adults due to the high prevalence of polypharmacy in this population. Age-related changes in pharmacokinetics and pharmacodynamics also increase the risk of adverse effects. This fact sheet addresses key interactions and provides some management strategies.

Drug-Drug Interactions (DDIs)

Mechanisms

- *Pharmacokinetic interactions*
  - Absorption: Older adults have increased gastric pH. This causes less drug to be released from tablets and capsules. Older adults also have decreased gastrointestinal (GI) motility, allowing more time for drugs to be absorbed. These two changes have an overall net zero effect on drug absorption.
  - Distribution: Most psychotropics are highly protein-bound. Older adults often have reduced serum albumin levels and less muscle mass, leading to decreased drug protein binding. As a result, a higher proportion of the drug remains unbound (free) and active in circulation, potentially increasing drug effects and toxicity.
  - Metabolism: The activity of CYP1A2 and CYP3A4 enzymes declines with age (mnemonic: A for age), leading to increased drug levels of their substrates. In contrast, CYP2D6 activity remains largely unchanged in older adults.
    - Inhibitors: These reduce enzyme activity, leading to increased drug levels of substrates processed by the enzyme. When prescribing a medication with a known inhibitor, consider:
      - Using lower doses and titrating more gradually.
      - Choosing an alternative medication that is not metabolized by the inhibited enzyme.
    - Inducers: These enhance enzyme activity, resulting in decreased drug levels of the enzyme's substrates. When prescribing a medication with a known inducer, consider:
      - Using higher doses to achieve therapeutic effects.
      - Selecting a different medication not metabolized by the induced enzyme.
    - Even with dose adjustments, inhibitors and inducers increase the likelihood of adverse drug reactions due to the altered pharmacokinetics. Careful monitoring is essential when combining these agents.

Table 41: **Common CYP450 Enzyme Interactions with Psychotropic Medications: Substrates, Inducers, and Inhibitors**

CYP Enzyme	Substrates	Inducers	Inhibitors
CYP1A2	Clozapine, caffeine, olanzapine, melatonin	Omeprazole, smoking	Cimetidine, ciprofloxacin, fluvoxamine, grapefruit juice
CYP2C19	Citalopram, clomipramine, diazepam	Carbamazepine, rifampin, St. John's wort	Fluoxetine, fluvoxamine, omeprazole
CYP2D6	Aripiprazole, codeine, duloxetine, fluoxetine, haloperidol, metoprolol, paroxetine, perphenazine, risperidone, tricyclic antidepressants (TCAs), tramadol, venlafaxine	Rifampin	Bupropion, cannabidiol, duloxetine, fluoxetine, paroxetine, sertraline
CYP3A4	Benzodiazepines, carbamazepine, HIV drugs, lurasidone, methadone, quetiapine	Carbamazepine, phenytoin, rifampin, St. John's wort	Clarithromycin, erythromycin, fluvoxamine, grapefruit juice, ketoconazole, ritonavir

  - Excretion: Older adults have reduced renal and hepatic clearance. This means that more of the drug stays around.

CLINICAL PEARL: *All these pharmacokinetic changes reinforce the adage in older adults to "start low and go slow" in order to lessen the risk of adverse effects and drug-drug interactions.*

- *Pharmacodynamic interactions:* Additive or antagonistic effects on drug action.

Table 42: **Clinical Implications of Common Psychotropic Drug Interactions**

Medication Class	Example Drugs	Common Interactions	Clinical Implications
Antipsychotics	Aripiprazole, olanzapine, quetiapine, risperidone	CNS depressants, QTc-prolonging agents (eg. antiarrhythmics, macrolides)	Enhanced sedation, metabolic syndrome, risk of arrhythmias
Benzodiazepines	Clonazepam, diazepam, lorazepam	Central nervous system (CNS) depressants (eg, opioids, alcohol), CYP3A4 inhibitors (eg, ketoconazole)	Enhanced sedation, fall risk, respiratory depression
MAOIs	Phenelzine, selegiline, tranylcypromine	SSRIs, SNRIs, TCAs, tyramine-rich foods	Serotonin syndrome, hypertensive crisis
Mood Stabilizers	Lamotrigine, lithium, valproate	Angiotensin-converting enzyme inhibitors, antipsychotics, diuretics, NSAIDs, SSRIs	Increased toxicity (lithium), hepatotoxicity (valproate), serious skin reactions (lamotrigine with valproate)
SNRIs	Duloxetine, venlafaxine	Anticoagulants, antihypertensives, NSAIDs, other SNRIs/SSRIs	Bleeding risk, hyponatremia, increased blood pressure, serotonin syndrome, urinary retention (duloxetine)
SSRIs	Citalopram, escitalopram, sertraline	Anticoagulants, antiplatelet agents, anti-psychotics, NSAIDs, other SSRIs and SNRIs	Hyponatremia, increased bleeding risk, serotonin syndrome, QTc prolongation (citalopram)
TCAs	Amitriptyline, nortriptyline	Anticholinergics, antihistamines, CNS depressants, MAOIs	Cardiac condition disturbances, CNS depression, enhanced anticholinergic effects, falls, hypertensive crisis

Specific Drug-Drug Interactions

Antidepressants

- *Selective serotonin reuptake inhibitors/Selective norepinephrine reuptake inhibitors (SSRIs/SNRIs) and nonsteroidal anti-inflammatory drugs (NSAIDs)/anticoagulants (Warfarin)*
  - Interaction: Increased risk of bleeding.
  - Management
    - Monitor INR closely with warfarin.
    - Consider alternative antidepressants such as bupropion or mirtazapine, which have a lower bleeding risk.
    - Educate patients on signs of bleeding.
    - Use gastroprotective agents (eg, proton pump inhibitors).
- *SSRIs/SNRIs and linezolid/triptans*
  - Interaction: Risk of serotonin syndrome.
  - Management
    - Monitor for symptoms of serotonin syndrome if a triptan is ordered for headache, though this interaction is uncommon.
    - Avoid co-prescribing with linezolid, an antibiotic used for vancomycin-resistant Enterococcus faecium (VRE), as it has monoamine oxidase inhibitor (MAOI) properties.
- *SSRIs/SNRIs and pain medications (tramadol, meperidine, fentanyl)*
  - Interaction: The FDA has warned that all opioids can increase the risk of serotonin syndrome when combined with serotonergic antidepressants.
  - Management: Avoid co-prescribing.

Antipsychotics and QTc-prolonging drugs

- *Interaction*: Increased risk of QTc prolongation leading to torsades de pointes, which can cause sudden cardiac death.
- *Monitor*: Electrocardiogram (ECG) regularly, avoid combining QTc-prolonging drugs if possible.
- *Medications*
  - The antipsychotics with the lowest risk of QTc prolongation are aripiprazole, brexpiprazole, cariprazine, and lurasidone.
  - While antipsychotics are often blamed for QTc prolongation, there are several medications prescribed on medical units that can prolong QTc. Be especially wary of combinations of antipsychotics and the following (Fazio G et al, *World J Cardiol* 2013;5(4):87-93):
    - Antibiotics
      - Macrolides: Azithromycin, clarithromycin, erythromycin
      - Fluoroquinolones: Ciprofloxacin, levofloxacin, moxifloxacin

Medication & Neuromodulation

    - Antifungals: Fluconazole, itraconazole, ketoconazole, voriconazole
    - Antivirals: Nelfinavir
    - Antiarrhythmics
      - Class IA antiarrhythmics: Quinidine, procainamide, disopyramide
      - Class III: Amiodarone, sotalol, dofetilide
    - Antiemetics
      - Phenothiazines: Prochlorperazine, promethazine. These meds have intrinsic antipsychotic properties and can also prolong the QTc interval.
      - 5-HT3 receptor antagonists: Ondansetron, granisetron, dolasetron
    - Antihistamines: Diphenhydramine, hydroxyzine
    - Certain anticancer medications: Tamoxifen
    - Certain diuretics: Furosemide
    - Opioids: Methadone at higher doses can significantly prolong QTc intervals.
  - Management
    - If an alternative medication is not suitable, consider ordering daily ECGs to monitor QTc intervals, placing the patient on telemetry when using medications with a high risk of QTc prolongation (such as intravenous haloperidol), and/or seeking cardiology clearance.
    - Ensure that magnesium levels are above two, as this can help reduce the risk of torsades de pointes. Additionally, it is recommended to maintain all electrolyte levels within normal ranges.
    - Discontinue the antipsychotic if QTc intervals exceed 500 ms or if there is an increase of more than 60 ms from baseline, unless cardiology has cleared the patient.

Benzodiazepines and opioids

- *Interaction*: Increased risk of respiratory depression, including sleep apnea, and sedation.
- *Management*
  - Avoid concurrent use, if possible.
  - Use the lowest effective doses.
  - Monitor closely for signs of respiratory depression (eg, respiratory rate < 12, oxygen desaturations, and shortness of breath with use of accessory muscles).

Mood stabilizers and other medications

- *Lithium and NSAIDs/ACE inhibitors/diuretics*
  - Interaction: Increased lithium levels, risk of toxicity.
  - Management
    - Monitor lithium levels frequently.
    - Educate patients on symptoms of lithium toxicity (tremor, confusion, vomiting).
    - Consider alternative pain management (eg, acetaminophen).
- *Valproate and enzyme-inducing antiepileptics (eg, carbamazepine, phenytoin)*
  - Interaction: Decreased valproate levels, reduced efficacy.
  - Management
    - Monitor valproate levels.
    - Adjust dosage as needed.
    - Consider alternative anticonvulsants.
- *Clozapine and carbamazepine*
  - Interaction: Increased risk of agranulocytosis and bone marrow suppression.
  - Management
    - Avoid co-prescribing.
    - Monitor absolute neutrophil count (ANC) regularly.
    - Consider alternative medications.

Cholinesterase inhibitors and other medications

- *Cholinesterase inhibitors (eg, donepezil) and anticholinergics*
  - Interaction: Opposing pharmacological effects that can result in decreased efficacy of the cholinesterase inhibitor.
  - Management: Avoid anticholinergic medications and monitor cognitive function closely.
- *Cholinesterase inhibitors and beta-blockers*
  - Interaction: Increased risk of bradycardia.
  - Management: Monitor heart rate and consider alternative medications if bradycardia occurs.

Deprescribing Medications in Older Adults

Most older adults take more than five medications, making polypharmacy a significant issue in this population. Deprescribing is the process of discontinuing medications that are either potentially harmful or are no longer required. This can reduce mortality, as well as improve cognition and quality of life.

Case Vignette: *Mr. Schneider, an 82-year-old with mild cognitive impairment, multiple falls, and daytime sedation, has taken 10 mg diazepam nightly for insomnia since retirement. A medication review reveals possible sedation and fall risk due to diazepam, a long-acting benzodiazepine. Together with Mr. Schneider and his family, you plan a gradual taper (ie, a 2 mg reduction every 2–4 weeks) and explore sleep hygiene strategies. Over two months, diazepam is discontinued, and his fall frequency decreases.*

Rationale for Deprescribing in Psychiatry

Changing risk-benefit ratio

Over time, a medication's benefits can diminish or risks can escalate due to aging, new medical conditions, or changes in a patient's psychosocial environment.

Polypharmacy

Leads to drug interactions, increased side effects, and difficulty in managing complex medication regimens in older adults.

Sometimes, the best addition is subtraction

In some cases, the most effective solution for an older adult is to reduce unnecessary medications rather than add more. Many patients experience improvements just from simplification of their medication regimens. So, before prescribing a new medication, consider the following questions:

- Has the current medication's dose been optimized? Was the trial duration adequate? Is the patient adhering to the current medication?
- Is the new medication being prescribed to manage side effects of an existing medication?
- Is the new medication intended to address the same symptoms as an existing one?
- Is the current medication necessary? Is it still providing benefit?
- Can the existing medication be given at a lower dose or gradually discontinued?
- Can the existing medication be replaced with a nonpharmacologic alternative?

Implementing Deprescribing: A Structured Approach

1. *Regularly update medication lists:* Ensure that the medication list is frequently updated and includes all prescriptions, over-the-counter (OTC) agents, and supplements.
2. *Assessment:* Complete a thorough review of all medications, identifying those with a questionable risk-benefit profile, potential for drug-drug interactions, poor tolerability in older adults, and those that are no longer required.
3. *Choose the right time:* Avoid times of crisis or an acute phase of illness. Ensure that a strong treatment alliance is established before deprescribing.
4. *Introduce deprescribing to the patient:* Inform the patient about the reasons for deprescribing and the process. Discuss any anxieties on the part of the prescriber, patient, family, or clinical care team.
5. *Identify which medication to taper*: Collaboratively decide which medication to taper or discontinue. Consider the patient's symptoms and alternative coping strategies. Taper only one medication at a time.
6. *Develop and implement a plan:* Set a start date and the amount of taper. Reinforce other strategies for addressing symptoms. Advise the patient about expected and likely discontinuation effects, as well as their timing. Provide close follow-up and support, adjusting the plan as needed based on patient's response (Gupta S and Cahill JD, *Psychiatric Serv* 2016;67(8):904–907).

How to Choose Which Medications to Taper Off

Criteria for identifying psychotropics for discontinuation

- *Long-term side effects:* Prioritize the discontinuation of medications associated with severe long-term side effects, such as tardive dyskinesia (TD) with first-generation antipsychotics or cognitive impairment and even dementia with anticholinergics.
- *Age-related pharmacokinetics and pharmacodynamics changes:* Aging alters drug metabolism and sensitivity, increasing the risk of adverse effects. Highly sedating medications and those that are anticholinergic should be considered for deprescribing.

- *Drug-drug and drug-disease interactions:* Evaluate for interactions that may exacerbate underlying conditions (eg, anticholinergic medications worsening cognitive impairment; serotonin norepinephrine reuptake inhibitors [SNRIs] worsening blood pressure); or interact with other medications (eg, fluoxetine inhibiting the breakdown of carvedilol), leading to increased side effects.
- *Duplication and efficacy:* This is a big one. Discontinue medications with overlapping therapeutic effects (eg, dual antipsychotic prescriptions or a selective serotonin reuptake inhibitor [SSRI]/SNRI combination) or those that have not shown clinical benefit. Try to use medications that address multiple symptoms at once.

CLINICAL PEARL: *Tools such as the* ***Beers Criteria*** *(American Geriatrics Society) and* ***STOPP/START*** *(Screening Tool of Older Person's Prescriptions/Screening Tool to Alert to Right Treatment) help identify potentially inappropriate medications.*

Specific psychotropic classes (in order of consideration)

- *Long-acting benzodiazepines and Z-drugs (eg, diazepam, zolpidem):* Given the increased risk of falls, cognitive impairment, and dependence, review these critically.
- *Anticholinergics:* Used in treating Parkinson's disease, extrapyramidal symptoms (EPS), gastrointestinal disorders, incontinence, insomnia, and muscle spasms. They can worsen cognitive impairment or cause urinary tract infections due to urinary retention; blurry vision leading to falls; or extreme discomfort from constipation. Reduce or eliminate, if possible, especially if used to counteract the side effects of another psychotropic. More information is available at www.thecarlatreport.com/anticholinergicactivity.
- *Antipsychotics:* Used for a variety of indications beyond psychosis, (eg, agitation in dementia). They carry risks of metabolic syndrome, EPS, and cardiovascular effects. Consider deprescribing, especially first-generation agents, like haloperidol, that carry higher risks of TD and death in patients with dementia-related agitation.
- *Mood stabilizers (eg, lithium, carbamazepine, gabapentin, oxcarbazepine, valproate):* Can have significant adverse reactions in older adults. The most concerning are carbamazepine (drug interactions and neurological side effects) and oxcarbazepine (syndrome of inappropriate antidiuretic hormone secretion/hyponatremia).
- *OTC medications:* Easy to forget but ask about commonly used ones like first-generation antihistamines, decongestants, proton pump inhibitors, and "PM" sleep aids, several of which contain antihistaminic and anticholinergic compounds. All of these can contribute to cognitive impairment or agitation.
- *Antidepressants:* While effective for major depressive disorder, some older adults may be maintained on antidepressants with a higher side effect profile (eg, paroxetine, tricyclic antidepressants, or monoamine oxidase inhibitors) or they may no longer need them. SSRIs/SNRIs, bupropion, or mirtazapine may be safer alternatives.
- *More information at* www.thecarlatreport.com/highriskmedsolderadults.

Challenges in Deprescribing

- *Patient anxiety:* Concerns about the resurgence of psychiatric symptoms can hinder willingness to reduce medications. Try slowing the tapering schedule and working on other strategies, such as psychotherapy, deep breathing/meditation, socialization, and exercise, to help manage symptoms.
- *Lack of guidelines:* Another significant barrier is the scarcity of robust guidelines and evidence supporting the safe discontinuation of psychiatric medications.
- *Perceived necessity of medications:* It can be challenging to change a stable regimen, especially in patients with complex, difficult-to-treat conditions. Consider a gradual taper, with more frequent visits to monitor progress, and engage the patient in discussions about the risks and benefits of tapering versus staying on their current regimen.
- *Patience:* Move at a pace the patient can handle and with their agreement. I had an older patient who took over two years to taper off clonazepam, but she eventually succeeded and subsequently experienced a significant reduction in falls (Gupta S and Cahill JD, *Psychiatric Services* 2016).

Neuromodulation for Older Adults

Neuromodulation offers an alternative to traditional pharmacotherapy for treating psychiatric disorders in older adults. This fact sheet provides information on various neuromodulation interventions, focusing on their application, effectiveness, side effects, discussion points for patients/families, and practical considerations for older adults.

Electroconvulsive Therapy (ECT)

- *Definition and mechanism:* ECT works by inducing a short (20–60 second) seizure under anesthesia via a brief electrical pulse.
- *Indications*
  - Severe depression, bipolar disorder (mania, mixed, or depressed), and schizophrenia, especially when rapid symptom resolution is needed.
  - In older adults, consider using ECT first-line for:
    - Depression in someone > 80 years of age
    - Depression with catatonic features
    - Depression with psychotic features
    - Depression with severe weight loss and anorexia
    - Treatment-refractory depression
- *Efficacy*
  - Highly effective for major depression, with response rates > 80% and remission rates > 60% in older adults.
  - Significantly faster response time in older adults (three weeks vs four weeks for meds) (Spaans HP et al, *Br J Psychiatry* 2015;206(1):67–71).
  - Can be a life-saving treatment due to its potent anti-suicide effect.
  - Older adults respond better than younger patients.
- *Workup*
  - Medical evaluation: Obtain a thorough history and physical exam to gauge overall health and identify any conditions that might complicate ECT.
    - Laboratory tests: Common tests include complete blood count (CBC), electrolytes, kidney function tests, liver function tests, and thyroid function tests to ensure there are no underlying issues that could cause problems.
    - Cardiovascular assessment: Electrocardiogram (ECG) detects any cardiac conditions that might make ECT riskier (eg, arrhythmias, ischemic heart disease).
    - Anesthesia evaluation: Order an anesthesiology consultation to review any risks associated with anesthesia and for airway assessment.
  - Consent process: Informed consent is needed. The discussion should include benefits, risks, potential side effects, and alternatives to ECT.
    - ECT can be a complicated recommendation to discuss with patients and their families due to stigma.
    - I will say something along these lines: "I'd like to talk about a treatment called electroconvulsive therapy, or ECT. It's important to consider all options, especially since the treatments we've tried so far haven't been as effective as we'd hoped. ECT is a procedure where controlled electric currents induce a brief seizure while the patient is under anesthesia. The seizures are carefully monitored and last only about a minute. The process helps to rapidly relieve symptoms of severe depression and other mental health conditions. It's one of the best treatments that we have in psychiatry. Almost 70% of people get better, and these are usually people who've had a lot of unsuccessful medication trials. It's also very safe in older adults. The mortality rate is about 1 in 70,000. The most common side effects are headache and some brief memory loss around the time of the procedure. ECT is usually done three times a week for 8 to 12 treatments in a specialized area with monitoring equipment, a nurse, an anesthesiologist, and a psychiatrist. If you decide not to pursue ECT, other options are continuing to make medication adjustments, psychotherapy, or other neuromodulation treatments like transcranial magnetic stimulation, though all are less effective. What are your thoughts?"
  - Baseline cognitive assessment: Conduct baseline bedside cognitive tests (eg, Mini-Mental Status Examination or Montreal Cognitive Assessment), to assess the patient's memory and other cognitive functions. This helps in monitoring for any potential cognitive changes resulting from ECT. Repeat cognitive tests periodically throughout the treatment course.
  - *Medication review*
    - Review and possibly adjust medications prior to ECT. In most cases, consider titrating off:
      - Agents that can increase seizure activity, such as bupropion, lithium, theophylline, and tricyclic antidepressants (TCAs).
      - Medications that can decrease seizure activity like anticonvulsants and benzodiazepines.

Medication & Neuromodulation

        - Medications that can prolong QTc intervals including TCAs and ziprasidone.
- *Protocol*
  - Administered two to three times a week for 6 to 12 sessions.
  - ECT is administered in an ECT suite equipped with an ECT machine, monitoring equipment to check the patient's vital signs (eg, heart rate, blood pressure, and oxygen saturation), and anesthesia equipment.
  - The team includes a psychiatrist (who administers the ECT and oversees the treatment), an anesthesiologist or nurse anesthetist (who administers the anesthesia and monitors the patient), and nursing staff (who assist with the procedure and post-procedure care).
  - Electrode placement
    - In ECT, the electrode placement can impact the treatment's effectiveness and the side effect profile.
    - Right unilateral (RUL) is generally considered less effective than bitemporal (BT) but is often used first in older adults because it is associated with fewer cognitive side effects. To achieve efficacy comparable to BT, higher stimulus dosages or more treatment sessions may be required.
    - Bifrontal (BF) placement is thought to balance effectiveness and cognitive side effects. Some studies suggest its efficacy might be comparable to BT but with potentially fewer cognitive side effects
    - BT is the most effective for rapid response and overall efficacy. It is used for severe cases of depression or when a fast response is critical. BT is associated with the highest risk of cognitive side effects, which can be particularly problematic in older adults.
    - I will usually suggest starting with BF or RUL and switching to BT if there is a lack of response by the sixth ECT treatment.
  - Maintenance ECT, or additional ECT after a patient has reached remission, effectively extends the initial response to ECT. I will recommend maintenance ECT for patients at high risk for relapse due to severe symptoms at baseline, rapid relapse after prior ECT treatments, or poor response to numerous medications and a long course of depression.
- *Side effects*
  - ECT is considered a safe procedure in older adults.
  - There are no absolute contraindications for ECT and no upper age limit.
  - Cognitive side effects: Anterograde and retrograde amnesia during the treatment course. There is no evidence that ECT causes structural brain changes, and most patient's memory improves following treatment completion (Kelly KG and Zisselman M, *J Am Geriatr Soc* 2000;48(5):560-566), though in some cases retrograde amnesia may resolve more slowly.
  - Cardiac side effects: Overall, considered safe, even in patients with heart failure. During the procedure, there can be arrhythmias, transient hypertension, transient bradycardia, and tachycardia, which can provoke ischemic changes, especially in patients with pre-existing heart disease.

Transcranial Magnetic Stimulation (TMS)

- *Definition and mechanism:* Uses magnetic fields to stimulate nerve cells in the brain. It is noninvasive and focuses on the prefrontal cortex to influence mood. It does not produce a seizure or require anesthesia.
- *Indications:* Major depressive disorder that has not responded to at least one adequate antidepressant trial.
- *Efficacy*
  - Moderate efficacy in reducing depressive symptoms, with improvement often observed after four to six weeks or sometimes longer.
  - Not recommended for depression with psychotic features.
  - May be less effective in older adults due to age-related structural brain changes such as brain atrophy which may weaken the intensity of TMS.
  - Response rates are 20%–50% lower than ECT (Galvez V et al, *Curr Psychiatry Rep* 2015;17(7):59).
- *Protocol:* Typically, five weekly sessions over four to six weeks. Each session lasts about 30–60 minutes. Unlike ECT, anesthesia is not needed, and TMS can be administered in an office.
- *Side effects:* Generally well tolerated; common side effects include scalp discomfort and headache. Rare risks include seizures. It is not associated with cognitive or cardiac side effects.

Vagus Nerve Stimulation (VNS)

- *Definition and mechanism:* Involves surgically implanting a device that stimulates the left vagus nerve through electrical impulses.
- *Indications:* Used as an adjunctive, long-term treatment for people with chronic or recurrent major depressive disorder who have not had an adequate response to four or more antidepressant trials.
- *Efficacy:* Data from the VNS registry indicate a positive benefit for VNS in older adults (McDonald WM, *Am J Geriatr Psychiatry* 2016;24(12):1130-1141).

- *Protocol:* Continuous stimulation; the device is typically activated one to two weeks post-implantation and adjusted as needed. Requires surgical follow-up and device adjustment.
- *Side effects:* Voice alteration, throat pain, and cough.

How to Choose Among Treatment Options

- *ECT* is considered the most effective option for severe and treatment-resistant depression, especially when there is a need for rapid improvement, such as in cases of severe suicidal ideation or psychotic features. ECT has superior efficacy to TMS.
- *TMS* may be chosen for patients with moderate to severe depression who have failed to respond to first-line antidepressant treatments but do not require the immediate response that ECT might provide or are concerned about the risks associated with ECT and anesthesia.
- *VNS* is usually reserved for chronic, treatment-resistant depression where other interventions (including medications, ECT, and TMS) have not worked. VNS is a long-term treatment strategy and may produce high response rates years after implantation.

Special Topics

Physical Activity and Nutrition in Older Adults

Physical activity and better nutrition can help prevent or slow cognitive decline and improve overall well-being. This fact sheet will provide information on the physical and nutritional needs of older adults.

Benefits of Physical Activity

- Regular physical activity reduces the risk of developing depression and anxiety and can enhance the quality of life of older adults.
- Physical exercise, such as senior walking groups, has been shown to slow cognitive decline and reduce the risk of dementia, eg, Alzheimer's dementia (AD).
- Exercise helps older adults maintain independence, prevent falls, alleviate pain, and manage or prevent chronic conditions like heart disease, diabetes, and osteoporosis.

Physical Activity Guidelines

- Ask your older patient: "How many days a week are you physically active? What kinds of things do you do?"
- According to the Centers for Disease Control and Prevention, older adults should aim for:
  - Aerobic activity: At least 150 minutes a week of moderate-intensity activity, eg, walking, or 75 minutes a week of vigorous-intensity activity, like hiking, jogging, or running. Older adults with chronic conditions or compromised health should be as physically active as their abilities and conditions allow.
  - Muscle-strengthening: Perform exercises involving all major muscle groups on two or more days a week.
  - Balance training: Yoga or Tai Chi can prevent falls. This is especially important for people with a history of falls.
- If these goals cannot be met, recommend that your patients walk for 30 minutes a day. Even just walking can lower dementia risk.

Nutrition Guidelines

Dietary approaches

- *Protein intake:* Prioritize to prevent muscle loss. The recommended intake is 1.0-1.2 grams per kilogram (kg) of body weight per day. So, for a person weighing 70 kg (about 154 pounds), the daily intake of lean protein should be 70-84 grams (g). This might look like the following:
  - Breakfast
    - Greek Yogurt (200 g): About 20 g of protein
    - Granola (1/2 cup): Approximately 4 g of protein
    - Hard-boiled eggs (two large): About 12 g of protein
  - Lunch
    - Grilled chicken breast (3.5 oz): Roughly 31 g of protein
    - Quinoa salad (one cup): Around 8 g of protein
  - Snacks
    - Cottage cheese (1/2 cup): Approximately 14 g of protein
    - A handful of almonds: About 6 g of protein
  - Dinner
    - Baked salmon (4 oz): About 23 g of protein
    - Steamed broccoli (1 cup): Roughly 3 g of protein
- *Carbohydrates:* Select from whole grains and avoid added sugars. Whole grains include whole wheat bread, pasta, or crackers; brown rice; oats; quinoa; barley; rye; and farro.
- *Fats:* Choose unsaturated fats. There are two types:
  - Monosaturated fats are primarily found in plant-based oils, nuts, seeds, and fish.
  - Polyunsaturated fats include omega-3 and omega-6 fatty acids found in fish like salmon, sardines, and trout, as well as in flaxseeds, walnuts, and sunflower seeds. Omega-3 fatty acids are known for reducing triglyceride levels, lowering blood pressure, and improving mood and possibly cognitive function.
- *Fruits and vegetables:* Critical components of a healthy diet.

Adequate fluid intake

Older adults generally require the same amount of water as younger adults, but they are more susceptible to dehydration due to a diminished sense of thirst and reduced kidney efficiency in conserving water. As a result, older adults may not feel thirsty even when dehydrated, making it crucial for them to consciously maintain proper hydration. Dehydration can lead to serious complications, such as renal failure, urinary tract infections, falls, weakness, and confusion. Encourage patients to drink 8–10 glasses of water daily, adjusted to health status and activity level.

Fiber intake

Important for digestive health and to prevent constipation. Whole grains, fruits, and vegetables should be part of daily meals. Fiber also helps manage blood sugar levels and lowers cholesterol.

Vitamin D, calcium, and vitamin B12

Critical due to their role in bone health and red blood cell formation. B12 absorption diminishes in older adults because of increased gastric pH, preventing its liberation from food. Supplementation should be considered if dietary intake is insufficient.

Antioxidant-rich foods

Berries, leafy greens, nuts, and seeds combat oxidative neuronal damage and inflammation.

Specific Diets to Recommend

During initial patient consultations, I emphasize the importance of diet in maintaining cognitive health. In addition to the well-established Mediterranean diet, I frequently recommend the Mediterranean-DASH Intervention for Neurodegenerative Delay (MIND) diet, which has shown promise in promoting brain health. To facilitate patient and family engagement with these suggestions, I provide informative handouts and direct them to reputable online resources, such as www.eatingwell.com.

Mediterranean diet

- *Description:* Characterized by high intake of olive oil, fruits, legumes, nuts, vegetables, whole grains, and cereals; moderate intake of fish; and low intake of dairy products, red meat, processed meats, and sweets.
- *Health benefits:* This diet is associated with reduced cardiovascular disease and mortality. It also supports better control of type 2 diabetes and helps maintain cognitive function. Greater adherence to the diet is associated with lower dementia probability, independent of genetic risk (Shannon OM et al, *BMC Med* 2023;21(1):81).

Dietary Approaches to Stop Hypertension (DASH) diet

- *Description:* The DASH diet emphasizes vegetables, fruits, whole grains, and low-fat dairy. It also incorporates fish, poultry, nuts, beans, and vegetable oils and limits sugary foods and beverages, red meat, and full-fat dairy. The standard DASH diet restricts salt to 2,300 milligrams per day, about the amount of sodium in one teaspoon of table salt.
- *Health benefits:* Primarily known for lowering high blood pressure, it also reduces the risk of heart disease and stroke (Siervo M et al, *Br J Nutr* 2015;113(1):1–15).

MIND diet

- The MIND diet (see "Table 43: MIND Diet for Brain Health") is a nutritional framework developed to lower the risk of dementia and declining brain health in late-life. It combines elements from the Mediterranean and DASH diets, while focusing on foods that impact brain health.
- *Health benefits*
  - Cognitive health: The MIND diet has been associated with slower cognitive decline. Studies have found that rigorously adhering to the MIND diet may reduce a person's risk of developing AD by as much as 30%–50% (McEvoy CT et al, *J Am Geriatr Soc* 2017;65(8):1857–1862; Morris MC et al, Alzheimer's Dement 2015;11(9):1007–1014).
  - Heart health: While targeted at brain health, the MIND diet also includes foods that are good for the heart, potentially lowering the risk of cardiovascular conditions.

Table 43: **MIND Diet for Brain Health**

Category	Recommendations	Key Benefits
Beans	More than 3 servings per week	High in fiber and protein, low in calories and fat, making them heart- and brain-healthy
Berries	2 or more servings per week (eg, blueberries, strawberries)	High in flavonoids, which are associated with slower cognitive decline (Devore EE et al, *Ann Neurol* 2012;72(1):135–143)
Butter and Margarine	Less than 1 tablespoon daily	High saturated fat intake contributes to vascular dysfunction and cognitive decline
Cheese	Limit to 1 serving per week	High in saturated fats; excessive intake linked to adverse vascular effects
Fried/Fast Food	Less than 1 serving per week	High in trans and saturated fats; linked to increased inflammation, oxidative stress, and cognitive decline
Fish	At least 1 serving per week	Rich in omega-3 fatty acids, which support brain health and reduce inflammation

(table continues)

Table 43: **MIND Diet for Brain Health** *(continued)*

Category	Recommendations	Key Benefits
Green Leafy Vegetables	At least 6 servings per week (eg, spinach, kale, salad greens)	High in vitamins and minerals; linked to reduced β-amyloid buildup and reduced AD pathology (Agarwal P et al, *Neurology* 2023;100(22):e2259–e2268)
Nuts	5 servings per week	Contain healthy fats, fiber, and antioxidants; linked to better cognitive performance, particularly walnuts (Theodore LE et al, Adv Nutr 2021;12(3):777–792)
Olive Oil	Use as the main cooking oil	Rich in monounsaturated fats; associated with reduced risk of heart disease and cognitive decline
Other Vegetables	More than 1 serving per day	Rich in nutrients and antioxidants that support overall brain health
Pastries and Sweets	Less than 5 servings per week	High in refined sugars and unhealthy fats, which promote inflammation and insulin resistance
Poultry	2 servings per week	Lean protein source; less saturated fat compared to red meats
Red Meats	Less than 4 servings per week	High consumption is associated with increased risk of cognitive decline and heart disease
Whole Grains	3 or more servings per day	High in fiber, which supports heart and brain health by reducing inflammation and improving vascular function

Weight Loss

- Poor nutrition and weight loss can cause frailty, which in turn can lead to falls, loss of independence, and long-term care placement. It is very difficult for older adults to recover from frailty, so it is best to address it early.
- Interventions
  - Significant or rapid weight loss may be due to malignancy, patients should be referred urgently to primary care for a comprehensive evaluation.
  - Evaluate for depression, financial constraints, bereavement, or difficulty preparing meals due to cognitive or physical limitations.
  - Identify medications causing anorexia, nausea, or altered taste (eg, acetylcholinesterase inhibitors, bupropion, eszopiclone, or selective serotonin reuptake inhibitors [SSRIs] and serotonin norepinephrine reuptake inhibitors [SNRIs])
  - Refer patients to a dietician for nutritional recommendations.
  - Recommend supplements (eg, Ensure® or BOOST®); incorporate nutrient-rich foods (eg, fruits, vegetables, whole grains, lean proteins, healthy fats) into meals; advise eating regular meals and healthy snacks between meals.
  - Increase support from caregivers regarding grocery shopping or meal prep. Another option is Meals on Wheels, which can help bring food to older adults with decreased mobility or cognitive impairment.

Complementary and Alternative Therapies for Older Adults

Complementary and alternative medicine (CAM) provides additional treatment options that may be appealing to older adults who are sensitive to medication side effects or prefer nonpharmaceutical approaches. Studies suggest that up to one-third of older adults use CAM. Despite its widespread use, the evidence supporting CAM in older adults is still limited. However, clinicians should be prepared to discuss CAM options with patients (Meeks et al, *J Clin Psychiatry* 2007;68(10):1461-1471). This fact sheet offers an overview of CAM therapies and practical guidance for integrating CAM into clinical practice.

Dietary Supplements

L-methylfolate

- *Description:* L-methylfolate is the bioactive form of folate, which is critical for neurotransmitter synthesis. Unlike folic acid, l-methylfolate crosses the blood-brain barrier directly and can deliver more active product to the brain.
- *Dose:* 15 mg daily.
- *Evidence:* May be particularly beneficial for individuals with methylenetetrahydrofolate reductase (MTHFR) gene mutations affecting folate metabolism. Add it to an antidepressant to augment its effect.
- *Side effects:* Very well tolerated.

Omega-3 fatty acids

- *Description:* Essential fatty acids have potential anti-inflammatory, neuroprotective, and energizing effects that may improve brain function and mood.
- *Dose:* 1–2.5 grams daily. Preparations comprised of at least 60% eicosapentaenoic acid (EPA) produce the most robust antidepressant effects (Sublette ME et al, *J Clin Psychiatry* 2011;72(12):1577–1584).
- *Evidence:* Some studies suggest benefits in mood improvement.
- *Side effects:* Mild, including fishy aftertaste, diarrhea, and gastrointestinal (GI) upset.
- *Caution:* Possible interaction with anticoagulants causing increased bleeding risk.

S-Adenosyl methionine (SAMe)

- *Description:* A compound involved in the synthesis of dopamine, serotonin, and norepinephrine.
- *Dose:* 400 mg twice daily, up to 800 mg twice daily.
- *Evidence:* Comparable efficacy to antidepressants in reducing depression. It has shown benefit for augmentation of partial responders to selective serotonin reuptake inhibitors (SSRIs) and serotonin norepinephrine reuptake inhibitors (SNRIs). SAMe also seems to positively affect joint health, another potential advantage for older adults. The evidence supporting SAMe's benefits for cognition in older adults is limited (Nyer M et al, *Psychiatr Clin N Am* 2013;36(4):577–596).
- *Side effects:* Nausea, diarrhea, headache.
- *Caution:* Risk of serotonin syndrome when combined with other serotoninergic drugs. It could induce mania in patients with bipolar disorder.

Vitamin D

- *Description:* Fat-soluble vitamin crucial for bone health and memory and implicated in mood regulation.
- *Dose:* 800-2,000 IU daily or 50,000 IU weekly.
- *Evidence:* Low vitamin D levels are linked to cognitive impairment and higher incidence of depression; supplementation may improve symptoms, with the strongest effect reserved for those with low baseline vitamin D levels.
- *Side effects:* Rare at recommended doses; excessive doses can lead to toxicity.
- *Caution:* Monitor serum levels of 25-hydroxyvitamin D [25(OH)D], especially in patients with renal issues.

Herbal Remedies

Ginkgo biloba

- *Description:* Ginkgo is one of the most widely used herbal products for cognitive impairment. It is thought to work by way of its antioxidant and anti-inflammatory properties.
- *Dose:* The recommended dose is 120 mg twice daily.
- *Evidence:* Studies have yielded inconsistent, though mostly negative, results. A large randomized controlled trial concluded that ginkgo did not significantly reduce the incidence of dementia or Alzheimer's disease in older adults (Snitz BE et al, *JAMA* 2009;302(24):2663-70). As a result, I do not recommend its routine use.
- *Side effects:* Common side effects include gastrointestinal symptoms, headache, nausea, and vomiting.
- *Caution:* Ginkgo biloba has platelet inhibitory actions, which can increase the risk of bleeding, especially in patients taking anticoagulants or antiplatelet medications. This can lead to serious adverse events like hemorrhages.

St. John's wort (SJW)

- *Description:* Used for mild to moderate depression.
- *Dose:* 600–1200 mg/day, with 300 mg taken three times daily as the best studied and most commonly recommended regimen.
- *Evidence:* Some studies in older adults show benefits comparable to standard antidepressants like fluoxetine but with fewer side effects (Nyer M et al, *Psychiatr Clin N Am* 2013).
- *Side effects:* Photosensitivity, GI disturbances.
- *Caution:* SJW causes many drug interactions via induction of CYP3A4 and CYP2C9. This is a major concern in older adults and could decrease effectiveness of estrogens, immunosuppressants, some antiarrhythmics, some antihypertensives, some antiretrovirals, statins, warfarin, and other medications. The combination of SJW with serotonergic antidepressants can also result in serotonin syndrome and is not recommended.

Physical Therapies

Acupuncture

- *Description:* Traditional Chinese medicine technique involving needle insertion to help regulate life energy or "qi."
- *Evidence:* A meta-analysis showed a reduction in late-life depressive symptoms when acupuncture was used with or without antidepressants (Cai W et al, *Geriatr Nurs* 2023;51:215-221), but overall, the quality of the evidence for acupuncture is generally low.
- *Session duration:* 20–30 minutes, one to two times per week.
- *Side effects:* Minimal, occasional bruising or soreness.
- *Caution:* Ensure sterile technique to prevent infections.

Exercise

- *Description:* Regular physical activity, including aerobic and resistance training. See the fact sheet "Physical Activity and Nutrition in Older Adults" [page 166].
- *Evidence:* Supports the reduction of mild to moderate depressive symptoms. Exercise is beneficial for cognitive and physical health. Supervised exercise groups may be preferable to solo workouts (Nyer M et al, *Psychiatr Clin N Am* 2013).
- *Recommendations:* At least 150 minutes a week of moderate-intensity activity, such as walking, or 75 minutes a week of vigorous-intensity activity, as tolerated.
- *Side effects:* Low risk; may include muscle soreness or fatigue.
- *Caution:* Tailor intensity to the individual's physical capabilities and health status.

Tai Chi

- *Description:* A gentle form of martial arts focusing on slow, controlled movements and breath.
- *Evidence:* Shown to reduce stress, improve mood and physical functioning, and potentially decrease inflammatory markers in older adults (Lavretsky H et al, *Am J Geriatr Psychiatry* 2011;19(10):839–850). Tai Chi also helps with balance and fall reduction.
- *Session duration:* Classes typically last 45–60 minutes, one to two times per week.
- *Side effects:* Very safe, low risk of injury.
- *Caution:* Ensure exercises are appropriate to the individual's balance and mobility levels.

Mind-Body Practices

Meditation and spirituality

- *Description:* Practices to enhance mindfulness or spiritual engagement include individual or group work, prayer, and participation in religious services.
- *Evidence:* Can provide significant psychological comfort, reduce stress, and improve overall well-being.
- *Session duration:* Daily practice, duration varies according to individual preference and capability.
- *Side effects:* Generally safe; some may experience increased anxiety, especially if there is a history of trauma.
- *Caution:* Provide support in finding appropriate spiritual or meditative paths that align with the older adults' beliefs and comfort levels.

Mindful yoga

- *Description:* Combines physical postures, breathing exercises, meditation, and mindfulness-based stress reduction.
- *Evidence:* Mindful yoga may improve the mental and physical health of older adults with depression. The beneficial aspects of mindful yoga include calmness, being nonjudgmental, letting go, and seizing the day (Lee KC et al, *J Psychiatr Ment Health Nurs* 2019;26(3-4):87–100).
- *Session duration:* 60–90 minutes, one to three times per week.
- *Side effects:* Risk of injury if not properly supervised.
- *Caution:* Adjustments may be necessary for physical limitations.

Creative Therapies

Music therapy/art therapy

- *Description:* Use of art or music by a therapist to address emotional and cognitive needs.
- *Evidence:* Can improve mood, reduce anxiety, and enhance social interaction.
- *Session duration:* Typically, 30–60 minutes, one to two times per week.
- *Side effects:* Very safe; no significant side effects.
- *Caution:* Treatment should be conducted by certified therapists, preferably in a group setting, to ensure benefits and social interaction.

Clinical Integration

Initial evaluation

Assess CAM Usage

- Given the widespread use of CAM, start conversations to understand each patient's current and past interactions with CAM treatments.
- "Are you currently using any vitamins, supplements, herbal medicines, or other treatments for your mental health?"
- "Have you previously tried any alternative therapies to manage your symptoms?"
- "Would you be interested in exploring nonpharmacological options like exercise or meditation to help you feel better?"

Risk/benefit discussion

Evaluating Evidence and Safety

- Discuss the limited but growing scientific evidence supporting certain CAM therapies.
- Emphasize safety and efficacy, noting that while some CAM options have substantial backing (eg, St. John's Wort, exercise), others might lack rigorous testing.
- Highlight that CAM can be used as monotherapy for managing mild symptoms but should serve as an adjunct to conventional therapies in cases of moderate to severe symptoms.

Potential interactions and contraindications

Carefully review the potential for drug interactions and contraindications, particularly with herbal supplements, as patients may mistakenly assume that they are safer than prescription medications. This can lead to unintended side effects or reduced effectiveness of prescribed treatments.

Caregiver Stress and Burnout

Caregiver burnout occurs when a caregiver's physical health or emotional well-being is compromised because of the stress of caring for someone with significant needs. This occurs when caregivers do not receive sufficient support, overextend themselves with too many tasks and responsibilities, or fail to adequately care for their own well-being. This fact sheet outlines what you can do to assess and help address caregiver stress and burnout in elder care.

Why is Elder Care Taxing?

- *Physical demands:* Care tasks can be physically strenuous, especially when the older adult has mobility issues or requires help with basic activities of daily living, such as bathing, dressing, or toileting. Many caregivers are older themselves and can struggle to assist in these situations.
- *Emotional toll:* Continuous care for older adults with chronic illnesses or dementia can be emotionally draining, especially for those who have no respite or relief.
- *Isolation:* Many caregivers experience social isolation because of diminished support systems. They also might have to give up their own hobbies or leisure time in order to provide care.
- *Financial strain:* Caregiving is often unpaid. It can create further financial burden for adult caregivers due to reduced hours or missed time from work.
- *Grief and loss:* Watching the decline of a loved one can cause grief and sorrow, especially as that person requires more assistance with routine tasks or begins to lose their core memories.

Clinician's Checklist

- Conduct regular check-ins with caregivers during each visit to assess their well-being and connect them with appropriate resources. This practice is crucial not only for the caregivers' health but is also vital for patient care. Burned-out caregivers might neglect the patient's essential needs, such as food, medication, and hygiene. Caregiver burnout also increases the risk of errors and, in severe cases, leads to aggression or abuse. Regular caregiver assessments help prevent these serious consequences, safeguarding both the caregiver's and the patient's health.
- Questions and comments for caregivers
  - "Up to 30% of caregivers become depressed. Are you noticing any signs of depression or burnout?"
  - "Have you observed any changes in your own health or well-being?"
  - "How are you taking care of yourself?"
  - "Would you ever consider joining a caregiver support group or talking with a counselor?"

Signs It Is Time to Seek Help

Recommend that caregivers seek help at the first sign of any symptom of burnout syndrome. This condition is characterized by four dimensions.

1. *Emotional exhaustion:* Overwhelming fatigue, increased irritability or anger, withdrawal from activities.
2. *Depersonalization:* Adoption of an indifferent, impersonal, and even cynical attitude toward the patient.
3. *Reduction of personal fulfillment*: Perception of care as negative or ineffective (Alves LCS et al, *Dement Neuropsychol* 2019;13(4):415-421).
4. *Physical symptoms:* Headaches, stomachaches, difficulty falling or staying asleep, other stress related physical issues.

Interventions

Mental health treatment

- *Description:* Caregivers have a high rate of developing psychiatric disorders, including depression and anxiety. If signs are present, refer the caregiver to another mental health care clinician for psychotherapy and, potentially, medication management.
- *Effectiveness:* Regular sessions and psychotropic medications alleviate symptoms of depression and anxiety, improve stress management, and address burnout.

Mindfulness-based stress reduction (MBSR)

- *Description:* MBSR involves structured programs that incorporate mindfulness meditation to help individuals focus on the present moment and develop a nonjudgmental awareness of their thoughts, emotions, and bodily sensations.
- *Effectiveness:* Research shows that MBSR reduces stress, anxiety, and depression among caregivers, enhancing their overall quality of life and ability to provide care.

Psychoeducation

- The Alzheimer's Association has a 24/7 helpline, support groups, and information for caregivers on what to expect (https://www.alz.org/help-support/caregiving).

- General recommendations for caregivers:
  - Schedule regular checkups with your primary care physician.
  - Incorporate physical activity into your routine.
  - Adopt a healthy diet, such as the Mediterranean or MIND diet.
  - Practice relaxation techniques and take regular breaks.

Respite care

- *Description:* Respite care services including adult day programs offer temporary relief to caregivers, allowing them time to rest and attend to personal needs. Respite can be provided through in-home care services or at short-term care facilities.
- *Effectiveness:* Regular breaks prevent caregiver exhaustion and burnout, supporting sustained caregiving efforts over longer periods.

CLINICAL PEARL: *Many caregivers feel guilty about using respite services or believe that the services will not provide the same quality of care as the patient receives at home. I will remind the caregiver that the best way to take care of the patient is for them to take care of themselves. I will also state that respite will never match the one-on-one care the patient receives at home but can provide "good enough" service.*

Support groups and counseling

- *Description:* Support groups and counseling are valuable interventions for caregivers. Support groups offer a communal space for sharing experiences, emotional support, and practical advice. Counseling provides a more personalized approach to address emotional and psychological challenges.
- *Effectiveness:*
  - Both interventions can mitigate feelings of isolation and reduce stress associated with caregiving responsibilities.
  - Support groups specifically offer:
    - Emotional validation and empathy.
    - Practical strategies for managing caregiving tasks.
    - Opportunities for self-care and respite.
    - Information about helpful resources and community support networks.

Caregiver and Support Group Resources

- *Alzheimer's Association*
  - Offers specialized groups for caregivers of people with Alzheimer's and other dementias.
  - Website: www.alz.org
- *Caregiver Action Network (CAN):*
  - Works to help those who care for loved ones with chronic conditions, disabilities, or diseases, as well as those supporting the living needs of older adults.
  - The website has an extensive toolbox and a caregiver help desk staffed by experts who can offer free support to family caregivers.
  - Phone: 202-454-3970
  - Website: https://www.caregiveraction.org/
- *Eldercare Locator:*
  - Public service of the Administration for Community Living. Connects older adults and their families to services.
  - The website has a caregiver corner with useful links and resources.
  - Phone: 800-677-1116.
  - Website: https://eldercare.acl.gov/
- *Family Caregiver Alliance (FCA):*
  - FCA offers extensive resources and support for caregivers of adults with chronic or disabling health conditions. Online caregiver support groups that focus on family caregivers are also available.
  - Phone: 415-434-3388
  - Website: www.caregiver.org

Geriatric Psychiatry in the Nursing Home

Working in nursing homes presents unique challenges and experiences due to the complex mix of psychiatric, cognitive, and medical issues encountered among long-term care residents. This fact sheet highlights some of the specific aspects of this work, including interactions with staff, regulatory frustrations, and communication with families.

Epidemiology of Nursing Home Patients

Prevalence

- Approximately 1.3 million Americans, representing about 4% of adults over the age of 65, live in nursing homes (https://tinyurl.com/2dwcnbkp).
- The likelihood of living in a nursing home increases with age, with about 8% of people aged 85 and older residing in these facilities (https://tinyurl.com/4ehyrhuf).

Reasons for nursing home placement

- Reasons for skilled nursing facility (SNF) placement include management of chronic health conditions, cognitive impairment, functional disability, and post-acute care following surgery, significant injury, or acute illness.
- Another common motivation for transfer is the absence of family members or caregivers who can provide care in the community.
- Nursing homes provide end-of-life services for people with terminal illnesses.

Prevalence of psychiatric disorders

- Most people living in nursing homes have a psychiatric disorder.
- The most common diagnoses are:
  - Anxiety: Common, often related to both environmental and personal factors.
  - Dementia: Present in a significant number of residents, often accompanied by behavioral and psychological symptoms.
  - Depression: Highly prevalent, frequently misdiagnosed and inadequately treated.
  - Psychosis: Can occur in the context of dementia or as a primary condition.

Brief Assessment and Treatment of Common Nursing Home Psychiatric Disorders

Anxiety disorders

- *Assessment:* Inquire about excessive worrying and anxiety attacks. Rule out medical causes (eg, cardiovascular, respiratory, and thyroid disorders).
- *Treatment:* Use cognitive behavioral therapy (CBT) and selective serotonin reuptake inhibitors (SSRIs) or serotonin-norepinephrine reuptake inhibitors (SNRIs), starting at low doses. Avoid benzodiazepines due to the risk of cognitive impairment, dependency, and falls.

Behavioral and psychological symptoms of dementia (BPSD)

- *Nonpharmacological management:* Implement environmental modifications (eg, reducing noise, optimizing lighting, minimizing room changes). Encourage routines that include physical activity and social interaction. Use the DICE model (Describe, Investigate, Create, Evaluate) to identify and treat causes of agitation (Kales HC et al, *BMJ* 2015;350:h369).
- *Pharmacological management*
  - For Alzheimer's dementia or vascular dementia, consider risperidone, aripiprazole, olanzapine, or brexpiprazole.
  - For Lewy body dementia/Parkinson's disease dementia, consider reducing anticholinergics and dopamine agonists. Medication options include quetiapine, clozapine, and pimavanserin.
  - For frontotemporal dementia, consider SSRIs, second-generation antipsychotics (SGAs), or trazodone for agitation.

Dementia

- *Assessment:* Utilize family and staff reports alongside cognitive screening tools like the Mini-Mental State Examination or Montreal Cognitive Assessment.
- *Treatment:* Use cholinesterase inhibitors (eg, donepezil) for mild to severe disease and add memantine for moderate to severe cognitive impairment.

Depression

- *Screening:* Use the Geriatric Depression Scale short form. Be mindful that somatic symptoms like gastrointestinal discomfort or pain may mask an underlying depression.
- *Treatment*
  - Over 50% of nursing home residents are prescribed antidepressants. SSRIs (eg, sertraline started at 25 mg daily or escitalopram 5 mg daily) are preferred due to their more favorable side effect profiles.

– Monitor for gastrointestinal side effects and risk of hyponatremia.
– Consider psychotherapy, especially for mild to moderate depression or in combination with medication for severe cases.

Sleep disturbances

- *Prevalence:* Sleep disturbances are common in SNFs due to a combination of factors, including altered circadian rhythm associated with aging, comorbid conditions (depression, chronic pain), and environmental factors (ambient noise, disruptive roommates, uncomfortable beds).
- *Treatment strategies*
  - Medication optimization: Review all medications for their potential contribution to insomnia (eg, stimulants, diuretics taken late in the day, donepezil given at bedtime).
  - Encourage healthy sleep hygiene: Promote at least 30 minutes of daily exposure to natural sunlight to help regulate circadian rhythms. Ensure residents participate in physical activity during the day to promote better sleep at night.
  - Pharmacological interventions
    - Melatonin: Although evidence is mixed, it may be beneficial for circadian rhythm-related sleep disorders or mild insomnia.
    - Sedating antidepressants (eg, mirtazapine or trazodone) may be appropriate for patients with comorbid depression or anxiety.
    - Avoid medications with a high risk of dependency or adverse effects (eg, benzodiazepines) unless absolutely necessary for short-term use.

Nursing Home Reforms

Physical restraints

- Historically, physical restraints were used to manage behavioral symptoms in nursing homes. However, significant reforms have reduced their use, prioritizing safer and more person-centered care practices.
- Focus on environmental modifications and behavioral strategies to manage agitation and aggression. Medications should be reserved for when those measures have failed.
- In situations where safety is threatened and alternative channels have not been successful, the patient may require transfer to the emergency department for assessment and stabilization.

Misuse of psychotropic medications

- Due to the previous high use of psychotropic medications, especially antipsychotics, in nursing homes, federal regulations mandate regular reviews of psychotropic medications to prevent overuse. Despite its FDA approval for agitation associated with Alzheimer's dementia, this regulation also includes brexpiprazole.
- According to the Centers for Medicare and Medicaid Services (CMS) guidelines: Residents who are ordered psychotropic drugs must undergo gradual dose reductions and behavioral interventions, unless clinically contraindicated, in an effort to discontinue these drugs.
- While this can be beneficial in some cases, in others, patients may decompensate when long-term medications are reduced or discontinued.
- The regulations have been effective. However, while there has been a decrease in antipsychotic prescriptions for BPSD, there has been an increase in orders for mood stabilizers, which have even less empirical support for treating BPSD.
- If medication reduction or discontinuation is clinically contraindicated, clearly document the patient's diagnosis, plan, and the risks and benefits of psychotropic treatment, stating: "Clinical dose reduction of (medication) is contraindicated at this time due to high risk of psychiatric decompensation of (diagnosis) resulting in possible injury to self/others or need for hospitalization. Nonpharmacological interventions have been employed alongside medication management to support the resident's mental health. The care team will continue to monitor the resident closely and reassess the potential for dose reduction in the future." If there have been previous unsuccessful attempts to reduce or discontinue the medication, also mention these instances.

Working with Nursing Home Staff

Collaboration

- *Develop partnerships:* Build strong relationships with nursing staff, therapists, social workers, and families to create and implement comprehensive care plans.
- *Team meetings:* Conduct regular team meetings to improve communication. Otherwise, make it a priority to discuss complex cases with nursing staff and directors and seek their input when planning treatment.

Challenges

Lack of specialized training: Many SNF team members are not specifically trained to work with individuals with mental illness and may not have expected this as part of their duties. Most will greatly appreciate psychiatric input and involvement.

Staff education

- *Education on psychiatric conditions:* Teach team members about recognizing psychiatric signs and symptoms, understanding their manifestations, and employing effective engagement strategies.
- *Ongoing training:* Provide ongoing training sessions, such as lunchtime lectures, to enhance staff competency and confidence in managing psychiatric conditions and challenging behaviors.

Emotional support for staff

Acknowledge stress: Recognize the stress and emotional burden that caring for residents with mental illness can place on staff members. Provide appropriate support to help them manage these challenges.

Communicating with Families

Regular updates

- Keep families or proxies informed about the patient's condition and treatment plan, especially since many SNF residents lack medical decision-making capacity.
- Address concerns promptly and involve families in care decisions to ensure a supportive environment for the patient.

Family education

- Educate families about the nature of the patient's psychiatric conditions and the rationale for treatment approaches.
- Provide resources and support to help families cope with their loved one's psychiatric illness.

Psychiatric Consultation in the Medically Ill Elderly Patient

Consultation-liaison psychiatry focuses on psychiatric presentations in patients with medical and surgical illnesses. Consultants see patients in the hospital, as well as in specialized outpatient settings. The most common reasons for consultation in older patients are the five Ds—delirium, dementia, depression, decision-making capacity, and drug effects—which are covered in separate fact sheets. This sheet will provide guidance on conducting consultations and some other commonly encountered issues.

Approach to Consultation

- *Reason for consultation:* Consults are typically requested by the primary treating team. It is often necessary to clarify the consultation question. Do this by calling the team for background information to better understand where you can be most helpful.
- *Chart review:* Ascertain the medical or surgical illnesses leading to the patient's hospitalization and potentially impacting their mental health. Appraise the existing clinical data (eg, chart notes, medication lists, vital signs, laboratory results, and diagnostic imaging).
- *Psychiatric assessment:* Conduct a thorough psychiatric assessment. Obtain collateral history from caregivers and outpatient psychiatric clinicians. Nursing staff are frequently able to provide information on behavioral measures (eg, cooperativeness with care, amenability to medications, agitation, sleeping patterns, percentage of meals eaten, etc).
- *Neurocognitive disorders:* Since delirium and dementia are the most frequent diagnoses seen, always assess neurocognitive function by administering a Mini-Mental State Exam, Montreal Cognitive Assessment, or the Saint Louis University Mental Status exam.
- *Recommendations:* Write a detailed consultation note with targeted items for the primary team to implement. Include safety considerations, tests for further workup, medication suggestions if applicable, behavioral strategies, support services, and a follow-up plan. Involve families and caregivers in care planning.

Catatonia

Clinical features

Catatonia presents with a variety of symptoms, broadly categorized as motor, behavioral, and autonomic. The DSM-5-TR criteria for catatonia requires the presence of three or more of these symptoms:

- *Motor signs:* Immobility, mutism, stupor, posturing (maintaining a posture against gravity), waxy flexibility (initial resistance to being positioned), rigidity, or negativism (no response to instructions).
- *Behavioral signs:* Echolalia (mimicking speech), echopraxia (mimicking movements), stereotypy (repetitive movements), or agitation.
- *Autonomic signs:* Tachycardia, hypertension, fever, or diaphoresis.

Screening tools: The Bush-Francis Catatonia Rating Scale is the gold standard for diagnosis. Visit https://tinyurl.com/y4mzrbyv for an instructional video on its administration.

Etiology of catatonia

- *Medical conditions:* Autoimmune disorders (lupus or multiple sclerosis), endocrinopathies, infections, metabolic imbalances, neurological conditions (eg, encephalitis, stroke, traumatic brain injury).
- *Medications:* Adverse effects of antipsychotics, withdrawal from benzodiazepines or L-dopa.
- *Psychiatric disorders:* Mood disorders (major depressive disorder, bipolar disorder), schizophrenia.

Initial assessment

- *History and examination*
  - Detailed medical and psychiatric history.
  - Comprehensive physical and neurological examination.
  - Review of current medications and recent changes.
- *Laboratory and imaging studies*
  - Basic metabolic panel, complete blood count, liver and kidney function tests, thyroid function tests, and creatine kinase (CK).
  - Brain imaging (CT, MRI) if neurological causes are suspected.
  - Electroencephalogram to rule out nonconvulsive status epilepticus.

Management of catatonia

- Nonpharmacological interventions
  - Supportive care: Ensure adequate hydration, nutrition, and management of vital signs.
  - Environmental modifications: Provide a calm, quiet environment to reduce stimulation and agitation.

– Monitoring: Continuous monitoring of vital signs and mental status.

- Treatment
  - *Benzodiazepines:* First-line treatment for catatonia.
    - Lorazepam: Initial dose of 1–2 mg IV or PO repeated every few hours as needed. Rapid response within 30 minutes confirms the diagnosis, though delayed reactions also occur. Maximum total daily dose is 24 mg.
    - Response monitoring: Assess for improvement in symptoms after the first dose; if successful, continue and titrate the dose based on reaction.
  - *Electroconvulsive Therapy*
    - Indicated for patients who do not respond to benzodiazepines or when rapid improvement is necessary.
    - Highly effective for catatonia, particularly when it is severe or life-threatening.
  - *Other medications:* Diazepam 10–30 mg; zolpidem up to 40 mg/day; amantadine up to 500 mg daily, memantine up to 20 mg daily (Sienaert P et al, *Frontiers in Psychiatry* 2014;9(5):121083).
  - *Address underlying causes*
    - Medical conditions: Treat underlying medical or neurological conditions contributing to catatonia.
    - Medication adjustments: Discontinue or adjust medications that may precipitate catatonia, such as antipsychotics.

Managing Behavioral Issues on Medical Floors

Common challenges:

- *Aggression:* Physical or verbal threats or acts.
- *Agitation:* Restlessness, climbing out of bed.
- *Refusal of care:* Resistance to medical treatments or interventions.
- *Wandering:* Moving aimlessly or attempting to leave the hospital.

Strategies

- *Assessment*
  - Identify triggers such as pain, discomfort, infections, medication side effects, or environmental factors, like noise or nighttime interruptions.
  - Rule out medical causes of behavioral changes, like metabolic imbalances or infections.
- *One-to-one observation*
  - Implement one-to-one observation or a safety sitter for patients who are at high risk of harming themselves or others or those with severe agitation that cannot be managed otherwise.
  - Have a low threshold for increasing the patient's level of observation as there are many ways patients can harm themselves on medical units due to the presence of cords, tubes, IV needles, and other means.
- *Nonpharmacological interventions*
  - Minimize noise and ensure adequate lighting.
  - Use calming sounds and familiar objects to create a soothing environment.
  - Provide activities to distract the patient, such as puzzles, books, or music.
  - Train staff to manage acute agitation or aggression by using a calm tone, maintaining a nonthreatening posture, and redirecting the patient's attention.
  - For refusal of care, consider assessing decision-making capacity.
- *Psychosocial interventions*
  - Involve family members to provide emotional support and engagement. Family at bedside can be a soothing and orienting presence for patients.
  - Utilize social workers, chaplains, and patient advocates to address psychosocial needs.
  - Psychologists can help develop behavioral plans for particularly challenging patients and address unmet emotional needs.
- *Pharmacological interventions*
  - Indications for medication: Reserve pharmacological interventions for when nonpharmacological strategies are insufficient or when the patient poses a risk to themselves or others.
  - Medication Choices
    - *Antipsychotics:* Use low doses of antipsychotics (eg, risperidone, olanzapine, quetiapine) for severe agitation or aggression. Olanzapine is available as an intramuscular injection for emergent situations. Monitor for side effects such as extrapyramidal symptoms and metabolic syndrome.
    - *Mood stabilizers:* Consider mood stabilizers (eg, valproate, carbamazepine) for patients with persistent behavioral disturbances, including disinhibited actions.

    - *Benzodiazepines:* Use with caution due to risks of sedation, falls, paradoxical agitation in older adults, and worsening cognitive impairment. Short-term use may be okay in some cases, especially for patients who cannot take high-potency antipsychotics due to prolonged QTc intervals, Parkinson's disease, Lewy body dementia, or other reasons.
    - *Monitoring and side effects:* Regularly monitor patients for side effects of psychiatric medications, adjusting doses as needed. For patients prescribed an antipsychotic, check frequent ECGs to monitor QTc intervals. Recommend maintaining magnesium levels greater than two and normalizing all electrolytes in order to lower the risk of torsades de pointes.

Pain Management

Under-treatment

- Common due to fear of addiction.
- The risk of addiction in older adults tends to be low, especially in individuals with no prior history of alcohol or drug use disorders.
- It is often better to prioritize treating pain to alleviate suffering, rather than risking under-treatment.
- Untreated pain in older adults can contribute to anxiety, cardiovascular complications, depression, impaired activities of daily living, increased risk for falls, reduced mobility, and sleep disturbances.

Options

- *Nonopioid analgesics*
  - Acetaminophen.
  - Use nonsteroidal anti-inflammatory drugs (NSAIDs) with caution.
  - Patches for localized pain: lidocaine, capsaicin.
  - Muscle relaxants: consider methocarbamol or baclofen; cyclobenzaprine has strong anticholinergic activity and should be avoided.
- *Opioids:* Use the lowest effective dose with regular monitoring.
  - Weak opioids: codeine; use tramadol with caution due to the risk of GI issues, cognitive impairment, fractures, seizures, serotonin syndrome, and higher all-cause mortality in older adults.
  - Strong opioids: morphine, oxycodone, hydromorphone, fentanyl, methadone, oxymorphone.
- *Adjuvant therapies*
  - Can be added to nonopioid analgesics and opioids.
  - Antidepressants (serotonin-norepinephrine reuptake inhibitors/tricyclic antidepressants).
  - Anticonvulsants (gabapentin/pregabalin).
- *Other therapies*
  - Physical therapy, occupational therapy, massage, acupuncture.
  - Biofeedback, cognitive behavioral therapy, pain psychology consultation.
  - Transcutaneous electrical nerve stimulation, hot/cold therapy.

Sexual Health in Older Adults

Sexual activity is an important part of health and well-being. It correlates with greater enjoyment of life in older adults. In a 2018 University of Michigan poll, 40% of people aged 65 to 80 said they were sexually active (46% aged 65 to 70, 39% aged 71 to 75, and 25% aged 76 to 80). About half of the men were sexually active and about a third of the women (https://tinyurl.com/3nufc9u6). Clinicians might avoid discussions about sex because they may unconsciously accept misconceptions about sexual activity in older adults.

Assessment of Sexual Health

- *Importance of open discussion:* Addressing sexual health begins with dialogue. Many older adults will not volunteer information unless asked.
- *Privacy:* Ensure a confidential setting for discussing sensitive topics, usually away from adult children or caregivers.
- *Approach:* Open-ended, respectful questions can create an environment where patients feel safe to discuss concerns.
- *Screening:* Evaluate potential problems including loss of libido, erectile dysfunction, and medication side effects. Ask about sexually transmitted diseases, which have been on the rise in older adults.

PRACTICE POINT: *I will often medicalize these discussions and say something like, "it's not uncommon for people to experience sexual side effects, while taking antidepressants. These can range from loss of libido to issues with performance. Have you noticed anything like that since starting [the medicine]?"*

Key Considerations

- *Aging:* Older adults may decrease sexual activity because of erectile dysfunction, vaginal dryness, arthritis, and bowel/bladder dysfunction.
- *Medical comorbidities:* Conditions like Parkinson's disease (PD), diabetes, coronary artery disease, and strokes can influence sexual health.
- *Medication side effects:* Medications, including those for depression, anxiety, and beta-blockers for hypertension, can impair libido and sexual function.
- *Mental health:* Most mental health conditions like depression, psychosis, or substance use disorders impact libido and sexual function.
- *Dementia and inappropriate sexual behavior:* Alzheimer's dementia and other forms of dementia may lead to changes in sexual behavior. Frontotemporal dementia and dopaminergic medications for people with PD can increase libido and disinhibited behaviors.

Management Strategies

- *Psychoeducation:* Discuss changes in sexual function with age, illness, and medications.
- *Tailoring treatments:* Depending on the cause, interventions may range from medication adjustments to ordering medications like sildenafil or referral to a specialist.
- *Addressing side effects:* Regularly discuss the potential sexual side effects of psychiatric medications with older adults and consider alternatives when needed.
- *Dementia*: Use behavioral interventions, and when required, medications to address inappropriate sexual behaviors. See fact sheet "Inappropriate Sexual Behaviors in Dementia" [page 144].
- *Safe sex practices*: Engage in discussions about safe sex practices with older adults. Many in this age group may not use protection due to a lack of sex education during their youth and the fact that HIV and other sexually transmitted diseases (STDs) were not widely recognized in the past.

Sexuality in Long-Term Care Facilities

- *Barriers:* Privacy concerns, staff biases, and concerns about consent.
- *Recommendations:* Enhance staff training and provide environments that respect the sexual needs and rights of residents.

Sexuality in Senior Communities

Increased opportunity: Today's older adults are more likely to participate in casual encounters and unprotected sex than earlier generations. Sexual activity might increase due to the availability of treatments for sexual dysfunction, growth of retirement communities, and the increased use of dating apps (Steckenrider J, *Lancet Healthy Longev* 2023;4(3):e96-e97).

Consideration for LGBTQIA+ Adults

Stigma: High levels of discrimination can make LGBTQIA+ (lesbian, gay, bisexual, transgender, queer [or sometimes questioning], intersex, asexual, and others) older adults reluctant to discuss sexuality or enter long-term care facilities.

Best practices: Use open-ended, inclusive language; avoid assumptions about sexual orientation; direct patients to resources like the services and advocacy for LGBTQIA+ Elders USA website (www.sageusa.org).

Legal and Ethical Considerations

Capacity and Competency Evaluations

You may be asked to determine decision-making capacity (DMC) in various situations, such as consent for medical procedures, for leaving the hospital against medical advice, or for other major decisions. In this fact sheet, I suggest an approach to evaluating DMC and what to do if you conclude that DMC is impaired.

Method for Evaluating Capacity in Older Adults

Assess cognitive function

- The Mini-Mental Status Exam or Montreal Cognitive Assessment are useful for a general assessment, but these tests are not specific for determining DMC.
- The aid to capacity evaluation is a standardized tool for DMC. It can be found at the University of Toronto Joint Centre for Bioethics (https://tinyurl.com/4bznbpp5). It takes 10–15 minutes to administer.

Respect the patient's autonomy

Involve patients in the decision-making process by using clear, simple explanations.

Evaluate a specific decision

Utilizing the four criteria for DMC as a framework, evaluate one specific decision (see table below).

Include patient and family

Family can provide insight into the patient's baseline decision-making abilities and preferences.

Engage a multidisciplinary team (if needed)

It can include neurologists, geriatricians, bioethicists, social workers, and legal experts.

Reevaluate frequently

Capacity may change over time, such as in people with delirium, so regular evaluation is essential.

Table 44: **Criteria for Decision-Making Capacity**

1. *Communicate a choice*
• The patient must be able to communicate their decision. This can be verbal or nonverbal, but it must be clear that the patient has made a choice. • Ask: "What have you decided?"
2. *Understand the relevant information*
• The patient should be able to understand the information provided by their team. This can be tested by asking the patient to summarize what they know about the situation and their options. • Ask: "Tell me what's happening." "What are your clinician's recommendations?"
3. *Appreciate the situation and its consequences*
• The patient must have an appreciation of the nature and consequences of their decision. This involves knowing the options available; the risks and benefits of each option; the potential outcomes of each choice; and the alternatives to each option. • Ask: "What are the pros and cons of your decision?" "Are there any alternatives?" "What could happen if you do or don't follow your clinician's recommendations?"
4. *Reasoning about options*
• The patient should be able to reason and use logic in making their decision. This includes being able to evaluate different options and to make a decision based on logical reasoning. The decision should be consistent with the patient's cultural, religious, and personal values. • Ask: "How did you come to this decision?" "What makes one choice better than the other?"

Capacity vs Competence

- *Capacity:* Determination is made by clinicians and is for one decision at one moment in time. Capacity is not a fixed state and can fluctuate.
- *Competence:* Legal determination made by a court. It refers to a person's legal ability to manage their affairs. It is usually used in the context of guardianship or conservatorship and is permanent.

Surrogate Decision-Makers

- When a patient lacks DMC, a surrogate decision-maker must be assigned to make medical decisions on the patient's behalf.
- If a patient does not have a designated healthcare proxy (HCP), family members can be used as surrogates. It is essential that the patient is protected from abuse or exploitation in these situations.
- If the patient has no HCP or family, in life-threatening situations, clinicians can make decisions on the patient's behalf; for nonemergent decisions, the court is often petitioned to assign an emergency temporary conservator or guardian based on the jurisdiction.

Elder Abuse: Recognition and Reporting

While thought of as uncommon, more than 10% of older adults may be victims of elder abuse (Lachs MS and Pillemer KA, *N Engl J Med* 2015;373(2):1947-1956). Despite this, the US Preventive Services Task Force does not recommend regular screening for elder abuse. So, often, it is assessed on an as-needed basis.

Identifying Elder Abuse

Elder abuse can manifest in various forms, including physical, emotional, or sexual abuse; financial exploitation; or neglect. Recognizing the signs of abuse is critical in initiating timely interventions. Here are some key steps to consider.

Initial assessment

- Evaluate the essentials, such as access to food, water, medications, and adequate shelter.
- Assess the patient's overall hygiene, nutritional status, and any unmet medical needs.

In-depth inquiry

Move on to more specific questions regarding the patient's social environment.

- Ask open-ended questions about the patient's daily life, relationships with caregivers, and any recent changes in their social or financial situation.
  - Focus on relationships with adult children or spouses, as they are the most likely to be the perpetrators.
  - Ask patients with dementia about finances, since they are most likely to experience financial exploitation.
- If you suspect abuse, it is crucial to interview the older adult alone so that they can share any concerns without fear of retribution.

Use of assessment tools

A structured tool like the Elder Abuse Suspicion Scale can help you systematically evaluate and document potential abuse (Yaffe MJ et al, *J Elder Abuse Negl* 2008;20(3):276–300). If you are not able to administer the scale, ask these questions.

- "Do you feel safe at home?"
- "Has anyone stopped you from getting things you need, like food, clothes, medications, or medical care? How about from seeing friends or family?"
- "Has someone not helped you when you needed help?"
- "Does anyone ever yell or curse at you?"
- "Has anyone tried to force you to sign papers or use your money when you didn't want to?"
- "Has anyone touched you inappropriately or physically hurt you?"

Nonverbal cues

- Body language and emotional state can offer clues to underlying abuse.
- Pay attention to nonverbal indicators, such as poor eye contact, withdrawal, anxiety, or hesitation to speak openly by deferring to the caregiver or potential abuser.
- In patients with limited ability to communicate either due to dementia or other medical conditions, nonverbal cues and physical signs may be the only sign of abuse.

Physical signs

Look for injuries or health conditions that may indicate abuse:

- Physical abuse
  - Jaw and cheekbone fractures are more likely to be sustained from a punch to the face than from a fall, which usually result in orbital or nasal bone fractures.
  - Multiple injuries in various stages of healing.
  - Signs of traumatic alopecia.
  - Unexplained injuries or fractures, particularly in atypical locations.
- Neglect
  - Evidence of inadequate or delayed medical care.
  - Evidence of undernourishment or dehydration.
  - Poor hygiene or unsuitable clothing (eg, not wearing a coat on a cold winter's day).
- Sexual abuse
  - Unexplained sexually transmitted diseases or genital injuries.

Managing Elder Abuse

Upon identifying signs of elder abuse, the following steps are crucial for management:

- *Immediate safety:* If the older adult is in immediate danger, prioritize their safety. This may involve hospitalization or arranging alternative accommodations to remove them from the abusive environment.
- *Reporting:* In most states, healthcare professionals are mandated reporters of elder abuse. Familiarize yourself with local laws and procedures for reporting to Adult Protective Services (APS) or law enforcement. When a report is made, an APS worker will visit the home and conduct an investigation.
- *Suggested strategies based on type of abuse* (Lachs MS and Pillemer KA, 2015):
  - *Neglect:* Optimize assistance at home, including finding other caregivers; educate the caregiver that the care being provided is inadequate; arrange for social work assistance to help with nursing home placement, adult day care, and other respite programs.
  - *Verbal abuse:* Refer the victim for social work assistance; educate the caregiver that the care being provided is unsatisfactory.
  - *Financial exploitation:* Stop the loss of resources as soon as possible; consider guardianship; alert banks and financial institutions to the victim's vulnerability; consider referral to local law enforcement.
  - *Physical or sexual abuse:* Refer the case to local law enforcement/district attorney; consider filing an order of protection with assistance of law enforcement; remove from the abusive environment; develop a safety plan.

Involuntary Hospitalization, Treatment, and Discharge

Involuntary treatment and hospitalization are critical components in managing older adults with severe psychiatric disorders who pose a danger to themselves or others and are unwilling to be hospitalized or receive treatment. This fact sheet provides a guide for clinicians in the hospital setting. It describes involuntary interventions and discharge of high-risk older adults from inpatient psychiatric units.

Risk Assessment and Documentation

Assessment

- The Joint Commission has mandated that all individuals evaluated for a mental health concern be screened for suicidal ideation with a structured tool such as the Suicide Assessment Five-Step Evaluation and Triage for Clinicians (SAFE-T) Pocket Card or the Columbia-Suicide Severity Rating Scale (C-SSRS). Patients should be classified as high, medium, or low risk for attempting suicide (Ryan EP and Oquendo MA, *Focus (Am Psychiatr Publ)* 2020;18(2):88-99).
  - SAFE-T: https://tinyurl.com/yt3hr2ez
  - C-SSRS: Access through The Columbia Lighthouse Project at https://cssrs.columbia.edu
- These assessments can help justify involuntary hospitalization; patients falling into the high-risk category will likely require psychiatric hospitalization, while those in the medium-risk category may require hospitalization.

Documentation

- Document specific behaviors, statements, or actions that indicate the patient's level of suicide risk (eg, suicidal ideation, plans, or intent).
- Clearly outline the rationale for any involuntary interventions, citing specific incidents, statements, or observed behaviors that necessitate such measures.
- Describe attempts to involve the patient voluntarily in treatment, including the patient's response to these efforts.
- Catalog relevant details provided by collateral sources, such as family members, outpatient clinicians, or others involved in the patient's care.
- Devise a treatment plan that addresses risk by commenting on treatment setting, level of observation, medications, therapeutic interventions, firearm safety, and follow-up care.

Criteria for Involuntary Psychiatric Hospitalization

In most jurisdictions, involuntary psychiatric hospitalization is considered only if the patient has refused voluntary admission and meets the following criteria:

- Presence of a psychiatric illness:
  - The patient must have a diagnosable psychiatric illness, not attributable to substance use, including intoxication or withdrawal, or antisocial personality disorder.
- At least one of the following:
  - Risk of harm to self:
    - Demonstrates suicidal ideation, intent, or behavior.
    - Engages in self-injurious behaviors that pose a significant risk to life or health.
  - Risk of harm to others:
    - Exhibits violent or aggressive behavior with a credible risk of causing physical harm to others.
  - Inability to care for basic needs (grave disability):
    - Displays significant functional impairment, such as being unable to secure food, shelter, or medical care, posing a risk to their survival.
    - Exhibits an inability to make rational decisions about personal welfare due to psychiatric illness, leading to potential harm or deterioration.

Considerations Regarding Involuntary Treatment

Legal framework

- When patients pose an immediate safety risk to themselves or others because of aggressive behavior, most states will allow for involuntary treatment over a patient's objections.
- Outside of an acute safety risk, for patients who are chronically refusing psychotropic treatment and remain at high risk, jurisdictions have varying statutes. Some require approval from a court, others allow for a hospital review process, before medications can be ordered.
- Understanding the specific statutes and regulations in your state is crucial for compliance.

Discharge of High-Risk Patients

Discharge of patients, particularly ones who have had involuntary treatment or hospitalization, requires meticulous planning and coordination to ensure their safety.

Criteria for discharge

- *Stabilization of acute symptoms*
  - Resolution or significant improvement of psychiatric symptoms (eg, no active suicidal ideation, reduced aggression).
  - Stable mood and behavior over a period of time.
- *Safety assessment*
  - Thorough evaluation confirming the patient is not an immediate danger to themselves or others.
  - Patient can perform basic care to manage their affairs.
  - Document use of a structured risk assessment tool to support the decision to discharge.
- *Support system*
  - Identify and involve a reliable support network (family, caregivers, community resources).
  - Attempt to confirm or arrange for a safe and stable living environment.
- *Multidisciplinary team involvement*
  - Engage a multidisciplinary team including psychiatrists, social workers, nurses, and occupational therapists.
  - Have regular team meetings to discuss the patient's progress, discharge readiness, and post-discharge needs.
  - Organizations may have a peer review or consultation process to evaluate high complexity patients prior to discharge. This can further support the discharge decision.

Discharge process

- *Comprehensive discharge plan*
  - Develop a detailed discharge plan outlining the patient's medical, psychiatric, and social needs.
  - Include specific recommendations for follow-up care, medication management, and therapeutic interventions.
- *Patient and family education*
  - It is often helpful to have a family meeting the day before discharge to marshal the patient's social supports.
  - Educate the patient and their family/caregivers about the discharge plan, including warning signs of relapse and crisis intervention strategies.
  - Provide written materials and contact information for emergency situations.
- *Medication management*
  - Ensure the patient has enough medications until the first follow-up appointment.
  - Provide clear instructions on medication administration and potential side effects.
  - Simplify medication regimens to enhance adherence in the days before discharge.
  - Recommend pill organizers or medication management systems for home use.
  - If there is a risk of overdose, medications may need to be stored in a safe or locked pillbox and dispensed by a support person.
  - Coordinate with the patient's pharmacy to set up medication delivery or pick-up.
- *Community resources and support*
  - Connect the patient with community resources such as home health services, adult day programs, and support groups.
  - Refer to organizations like the Alzheimer's Association or local mental health agencies for additional support.
- *Follow-up appointments*
  - Schedule follow-up appointments with mental health professionals (psychiatrists, therapists) within one to two weeks of discharge.
  - Ensure appointments with primary care providers and other specialists are arranged as necessary.

Additional Discharge Considerations

Suicide risk

- Have intensive follow-up and monitoring for patients with a history of suicidal ideation or attempts.
- For safety planning, include removing access to means of self-harm (eg, buying a locked medication box or a gun locker) and providing crisis hotline numbers (eg, 211 and 988).

Violence risk

- Coordinate with caregivers to manage potential triggers for aggressive behavior.
- Consider environmental modifications to reduce stressors and prevent escalation, important for patients with major neurocognitive disorders.

Grave disability

- Provide caregiver education regarding the patient's specific needs and how to manage emergencies.

- Connect patients and caregivers with community resources such as adult day programs, respite care, support groups, transportation services, and meal delivery programs.
- Offer referral to a case manager/social worker to coordinate services and monitor the patient's progress.
- Evaluate the need for assisted living or a skilled nursing facility, if home care is inadequate.
- Plan for legal and financial considerations, such as referral to an eldercare attorney for power of attorney, guardianship, and healthcare proxies.

End-of-Life Issues in Geriatric Psychiatry

You may be asked to consult on older adults who are close to the end of their lives. These issues are complex and sensitive and require that you understand the basics of hospice and palliative care. In this fact sheet, I provide an overview of these and other end-of-life issues, with recommendations for how you can help consult with the medical team.

Hospice and Palliative Care

Hospice care

- Hospice is indicated for patients in the last six months of life. It emphasizes pain and symptom management, psychosocial support, and spiritual care, rather than life-prolonging treatments.
- It is delivered primarily at home but also in hospice centers, hospitals, and long-term care facilities.
- The hospice care team includes hospice physicians, hospice nurses, social workers, chaplains/spiritual care providers, bereavement counselors, home health aides, and other specialists including mental health clinicians.
- To connect patients to hospice care, in the hospital, a consultation is placed to the service. In the outpatient setting, social workers or case managers can help link patients to organizations or centers that provide this type of care.

CASE VIGNETTE 1: *Mr. Cho, an 80-year-old man with metastatic lung cancer, is told that he has a few months to live. He has decided to discontinue aggressive treatments and transitions to hospice care to focus on comfort, pain relief, and emotional support for both himself and his family during his final months. Psychiatry is consulted to assist with anxiety management and to help him process his thoughts about dying. He starts supportive psychotherapy, which offers him a safe space to express his fears and emotions, while exploring meaning and legacy. Mr. Cho also starts taking mirtazapine for anxiety, insomnia, and appetite stimulation and PRN (as needed) alprazolam for anxiety attacks.*

Palliative care

- Palliative care focuses on providing symptomatic relief to people with life-impairing illnesses, as well as from pain.
- It aims to improve quality of life for both the patient and the caregiver/family.
- Palliative care is appropriate at any stage of illness and can be provided alongside curative treatment.
- Palliative care differs from hospice in that it is offered to patients with serious illnesses who have a life expectancy of longer than six months.
- Examples of such illnesses include advanced heart failure; moderate to severe COPD; chronic kidney disease, particularly for patients receiving dialysis; cirrhosis or other significant liver disease; multiple sclerosis and other neurological conditions; and HIV/AIDS.

CASE VIGNETTE 2: *Mrs. Thompson, a 78-year-old woman with advanced heart failure, was referred to palliative care due to debilitating dyspnea and fatigue, despite optimal medical treatment. A psychiatric consultation was sought to address fatigue, which was compounded by orthopnea, insomnia, and anxiety. To manage insomnia without compromising respiratory function, ramelteon was prescribed. It was also recognized that her anxiety intensified during episodes of dyspnea, leading to catastrophic thinking and further sleep disruption. The palliative care team worked collaboratively to optimize her cardiac medication regimen, as well as to challenge these negative thought patterns. With these interventions, Mrs. Thompson experienced some relief.*

Major Neurocognitive Disorder as a Terminal Diagnosis

- Major neurocognitive disorders, such as Alzheimer's dementia (AD) and other dementias, are progressive and incurable. Patients with advanced dementia have a life expectancy of one to two years.
- Increasingly, dementia specialists are referring patients for hospice care when they have reached a terminal stage of the disease with limited life expectancy and low quality of life.

Signs of end-stage dementia

- Impaired communication—less than six words a day.
- Reduced appetite and difficulty swallowing, leading to anorexia and weight loss.
- Incontinence.
- Recurrent hospital admissions due to pneumonia, urinary tract infections, or other causes.

- Trouble breathing.
- Motor changes such as inability to sit up, trouble walking, or difficulty smiling (Crowther J and Costello J, *Int J Pallia Nurs* 2017 2;23(10):502-510).

Treatment

Focus on symptom management; controlling pain and anxiety; managing symptoms of terminal delirium; maintaining comfort; and addressing the psychological and social needs of both the patient and caregivers.

CASE VIGNETTE 3: *Mr. Morgan, an 84-year-old man with advanced AD, is referred to hospice care due to his rapidly declining condition. He presents with signs of end-stage dementia, including minimal verbal communication, significant weight loss due to difficulty swallowing, and frequent hospital admissions for pneumonia. The psychiatrist involved in Mr. Morgan's care focuses on managing anxiety and terminal delirium with medications like low-dose lorazepam. The psychiatrist also provides emotional support to Mr. Morgan's family, helping them cope with anticipatory grief and guiding them in understanding his condition. Through regular consultations, the psychiatrist ensures Mr. Morgan's comfort and dignity are maintained in his final weeks.*

Delirium in the Hospice Care Setting

Prevalence

- Terminal delirium occurs in the last days and hours of life. It is sometimes referred to as "terminal agitation" or "terminal restlessness."
- It is the result of end-stage multisystem organ failure and other irreversible factors.
- The prevalence of terminal delirium is estimated to be as high as 88% in actively dying patients (Sutherland M et al, *J Hosp Palliat Nurs* 2019 21(5):430-437).

Workup

Usually very limited and should only be to help with symptomatic control.

Management

- *Nonpharmacological interventions:* Reorientation and other environmental measures will not be helpful. Instead, optimize the setting to enhance patient comfort by adjusting lighting, reducing noise, decreasing nighttime interruptions, allowing visitors, etc.
- *Pharmacological interventions*
  - Second-generation antipsychotics such as olanzapine or quetiapine are the mainstay interventions. If they are ineffective, haloperidol 0.5–1 mg orally or intravenously, repeated every four to six hours as needed can be used.
  - In terminal delirium, there is a much lower threshold to add benzodiazepines, opioids, or barbiturates to manage symptoms of agitation or restlessness. Some medications to consider when others have failed to help are:
    - Lorazepam 0.5–1 mg any route, with max daily dosage of 20 mg.
    - Midazolam
      - Loading dose: 0.1–0.2 mg/kg IV/SC, then repeated every 30 min PRN agitation
      - Maintenance dose: 0.02–0.2 mg/kg/h with max daily dose of 20 mg.
    - Phenobarbital
      - Loading dose: 50–100 mg IV every 10–15 min until comfortable
      - Maintenance dose: 60–800 mg divided over 24 h, with max daily dose of 800 mg. Used primarily for palliative sedation.

  (Source: Hategan A et al, eds. Geriatric Psychiatry: A Case-Based Textbook, Second Edition. Switzerland AG: Springer Nature Group; 2024)

Depressive Disorders in the Hospice Care Setting

Prevalence

Dismay is an expected part of the spectrum of responses during the dying process. Depressive disorders are common at the end of life, with an estimated prevalence of 24%–70%. Depression leads to decreased quality of life and may contribute to a desire for earlier death (Perusinghe M et al, *J Palliat Med* 2021;24(5):767-781).

Assessment

Though there is significant overlap between end-stage diseases and neurovegetative symptoms of depression, continue to utilize SIGECAPS criteria and screening tools such as the Geriatric Depression Scale (GDS) to make the diagnosis.

Management

- *Nonpharmacological interventions:* Supportive psychotherapy, music therapy, pastoral counseling, and spiritual therapy.
- *Pharmacological interventions*
  - Depressive disorders should be treated in order to minimize suffering, as well as to allow the patient to engage effectively with friends, family, therapists, or others at the end of life. With newer antidepressants, the benefits usually outweigh the risks.
  - Selective serotonin reuptake inhibitor (SSRI)/serotonin-norepinephrine reuptake inhibitor (SNRI): Sertraline 25–75 mg daily, escitalopram 5–20 mg daily, or venlafaxine 37.5–75 mg daily.
  - Mirtazapine 7.5–15 mg at bedtime.
  - Psychostimulants
    - There is a lower threshold at end of life to augment antidepressants with psychostimulants to potentially produce a faster response, though watch for worsened anxiety or irritability.
    - Consider
      - Methylphenidate 2.5 mg qAM or BID (AM and 1400), maximum total daily dose 20mg.
      - Modafinil PO 100 mg qAM, maximum dose 400 mg daily.

Anxiety Disorders in the Hospice Care Setting

Prevalence

- Estimates of the prevalence of anxiety disorders in the palliative care setting are 7%–13%, with significant anxiety symptoms occurring in 24%–48% (Atkin N et al, *BMC Palliat Care* 2017;16(1):69).
- Anxiety might manifest as constant worry, nervousness, tremors, difficulty sleeping, or increased muscle tension.

Management

- *Nonpharmacological interventions:* Relaxation techniques, supportive psychotherapy, spiritual counseling.
- *Pharmacological interventions*
  - Benzodiazepines (lorazepam, diazepam, alprazolam) as needed are a first-line or second-line choice.
    - Prescribe them in combination with an SSRI/SNRI (mirtazapine, sertraline, escitalopram)
  - Other medications to consider are pregabalin, quetiapine, olanzapine, and haloperidol (Atkin N et al, *BMC Palliat Care* 2017).